Tom's Law

How to Succeed as a Personal Trainer

Tom Law

OAM, Dip. Fitness

Contact the author:
tom@tomslaw.com.au
tomslaw.com.au

ISBN 978-0-6480300-0-3 (pbk)

Set in Linux Libertine

Dedicated to my wife, Margaret,
for allowing me to be me

Special thanks to: Donna Davis, Michael Glover, Brett Buktenica, Kimberley Healy, Deb Moor, Sally-Anne Stubbings, Shendelle Harrison, Marlene McDermid, Alastair McTavish, Gerrard Gosens and Monica Batiste for their advice, guidance and support and contributions while writing this book.

About the author

Tom Law came to Australia as a three-year-old, from Scotland. Settling in Geraldton, Western Australia, after finishing school he completed an apprenticeship as an electrician before marrying his wife, Margaret, and joining the Australian Army.

After 21 years of service in the Royal Australian Corps of Signals, and having been awarded an Order of Australia Medal for his services to training, Thomas went back to civilian life, working in his own business, then council and eventually managing a gym.

For the last 20 years, Tom has continued his education in the health and wellness field, and works today in his own fitness business, Tom's Law.

To contact Tom, please visit tomslaw.com.au.

Also by Tom Law

People and Places (2014)

Contents

Photos

The things Tom Law encourages you to do
are wide and varied all year through.
I've abseiled backwards and forwards too.
Seen beautiful sunrises of every hue.

We have run in the rain
Raced go-karts like kids again,
walked up and down Mt Mee,
flown across the ditch for a ski.

Raced through the tyres,
walked on high wires,
balanced on top of a six-metre pole,
played soccer and even scored a goal.

Been tucked up in a tractor tyre for a race,
then rolled at an astonishing pace.
Crawled under the net, propelled over a wall,
even went to a cowboy ball.

Rode our bikes, learned to snow ski,
stand up paddle board and surf in the sea.
Jumped the leap of faith, Mal was
    blindfolded too,
Played Commando Tennis with big balls,
had lots of laughter, and some falls.

The reason we keep coming back for more
Is exercise is fun when it's not a chore.

—Marlene McDermid

Foreword: Introducing Tom

Luke Howarth MP

The mental and physical rewards that come from participating in sport are widely sought after in the fast-paced, demanding and too often stressful environment that is life in the 21st century. So it's no wonder many people are trading in office work for sports coaching and personal training.

However, it takes a special kind of person to break through this now saturated industry – one who has entered the world of personal training (PT) not just for themselves, but to help others.

Tom Law's service began in the Australian Army and lasted a notable 21 years, which included a posting to the Special Air Service Regiment. He then joined the Pine Rivers Shire Council as an events co-ordinator.

In 2005, Tom left the council to start his own full-time business called "Breakout Adventures". The experience he gained in the military gave Tom the aptitude to work with corporate and professional sporting teams such as the Brisbane Lions AFL team, Sydney FC and Westpac Bank. Breakout Adventures was bought by Spectrum Health & Fitness, and Tom became the manager of this gym.

In 2006, in conjunction with the then-CEO, Tom started a new fitness program called Corporate Commando. Today, the session is just called Commando, and although Tom has left the gym, the business continues to thrive.

Now based in Redcliffe, but working in all areas of the Moreton Bay Region, Tom runs programs under the banner of 'Tom's Law', and regularly contributes to Moreton Bay Regional Council's outdoor recreational programs (including 'O Tag Fun Runs' and 'Spring in Your Step').

Before entering Parliament, I was proud to give back to our community as a volunteer judo coach at the Redcliffe Police Citizens Youth Club (PCYC). I know how much effort is involved in organising lessons and competitions, providing after-hours mentoring and helping students rise through challenges and levels (or belts, in the case of judo). Therefore, to say that Tom Law gives back to our local community is to say the least. He gives back – not just in time, but in effort, enthusiasm and incredible passion.

Tom was awarded an Order of Australia Medal for his services to training in the Army with the Royal Australian Corps of Signals. He was the Moreton Bay Regional Council Sportsperson of the Year for 2014, and he was awarded a Paul Harris Fellowship by Rotary International for his services to the community, specifically the Pine Rivers Charity Fun Run. He has a Certificate III and IV and a Diploma of Fitness qualification.

Tom and his wife, Margaret, have three adult children and live in Redcliffe, just across the road from Tom's favourite area to work out – Suttons Beach.

I applaud Tom for his career to date, and I have no doubt all his clients appreciate his hard work. His success and large following is testimony to his dedication to improving the health and lives of anyone who happens across his programs. I am sure the readers of this book will benefit from the years of experience and incredible passion that Tom brings to the industry.

Luke Howarth MP
Federal Member for Petrie

Why did I write this book?

I thought you might like to understand my motivation for writing this book before you read the contents. As a person involved in physical fitness from a very early age, it has been a passion of mine to keep myself as healthy as possible. I would like to see the world a lot healthier! I know this might seem like a comment from a Miss World interview, but it is true. A great deal of sickness is directly related to poor habits in exercise and nutrition. I see a lot of overweight and unhealthy people. It is a sad state of affairs and relevant authorities all over the world are attempting to address this health issue. I know we can help, even if only in a small way.

So back to the reasons why I wrote this book! I hope that those new[1] to the industry will benefit from my years of experience and may consider using some of my recommendations. Keep in mind that one of the roles of health professionals, as I see it, is to help people

---

[1]New to the industry does not always mean young people. I am aware of quite a few mature age people who have made the sea change to the health industry.

help themselves. The better we are at imparting our knowledge, the greater chance we have of achieving this.

I have observed fitness professionals over the years who would be much better with some simple coaching. "Being better" translates into having a good income stream, either working for someone else or yourself. It's true that some in the industry have professional development coaches, but many don't and would benefit from this addition.

It is not always possible or affordable when starting out to have the services of a coach. This book will provide you with good advice and practical solutions to some of the situations you will find yourself in, and go a long way to fulfilling the role of a coach.

Almost daily, I see fitness professionals working with clients in and around our local area, and their inexperience shows through. I see poor demonstrations, instruction by mobile phone, a lack of direct, appropriate and concise communication, and a general lack of professionalism. I have no doubt that the majority are well trained and educated in the ways of human anatomy and movement, but their customer service skills are sadly lacking.

My aim is that this publication goes some way towards stimulating discussion about how we, as a profession, go about our business, and that readers of this book learn from my experience and mistakes, and not only implement some of my suggestions but improve on them to suit their style of delivery.

I have been encouraged, by a number of people over the years, to write this book as a reference for those who are currently training to work in the health and wellness industry. The field we work in is fantastic. Together we can help reduce the burden of public health expenditure by contributing to a healthier society. The contribution we make in this area is already significant, but I am sure that in conjunction with other health professionals we can do more. If this book inspires you to be a better health professional, then I will consider that one of my aims in writing this book has been fulfilled.

I currently run my business from the Redcliffe Peninsula just north of Brisbane. I have been doing my sole operator outdoor group and personal training now for about eight years, having run a very successful gym before that. My name is well known in the area, we have a great brand and, I am very happy to say, a fantastic reputation locally.

This did not come by accident. I have worked hard and smart to achieve this, and to this day I continue to work in this way to maintain my business and knowledge in the industry.

So, here it is! I hope you enjoy this book, but more importantly, I know you will learn a lot from reading this. Together we can be part of the larger plan to help make your community a better one through good health and nutrition.

Tom Law
OAM Dip. Fitness

What will you get from this book?

At nearly every physical group training session, I tell my clients that they will only get out of the session what they are prepared to put in. This is not simply restricted to our field; I think it really applies to life generally. I want this book to work the same way. If you are willing to try something different and you want to be the best possible provider you can be, this publication will help. Of this I have no doubt.

I know that we are living in a very progressive and technological world. Today, I was told about the possibility of people being given an implant somewhere in the body that would perform the job of a personal trainer. Apparently, it is being worked on now. Nothing surprises me, and you will no doubt make up your own mind about these devices should they eventuate. You should always embrace new technology because most of it is fantastic and can make your job so much easier. Technology cannot do the job for you, so your skill set and experience will always count a great deal in how you conduct your business and how successful you will be. Success is measured in many ways, including personal satisfaction at a job well done. Your idea of success may be to be able to earn a decent living in the health and wellness field.

The field of the personal and group trainer has changed in many ways since I started in this trade. Most changes have been for the better, and I am sure that there will be more technical advances that assist both the trainer and client. I am hopeful and cautiously optimistic that despite the expected technical and electronic advances there will always be a place for the well-educated, gifted and dedicated personal and group fitness trainer. Keep up to date, make the changes and move with the times, but never substitute technology for good instruction, knowledge and personal attention to your clients.

This publication will give you an insight into how I operate my business, and how I believe we should all be grateful that we work in such a very positive industry. Like all professions, we are not entirely squeaky clean, and we have a few areas that could do with a polish or clean up, but I can tell you one thing for sure, the fitness industry in Australia is in a better state than it was years ago. Regulations, registrations, insurances and small claims tribunals have all helped to make our industry as good as it can be. The instances of gyms closing without any consultation with members, and taking all their fees with them may still happen on occasion, but the numbers are small now compared to days gone by.

Regardless of where in the world you are operating, you will find something beneficial from this book. I continue to travel, and I have visited gyms around the world. Although each country has its own subtly different way of doing things, we all have much in common and work towards the same goal: To help those in our community to be fitter, healthier and find the right balance in life for themselves.

You will get information in this book that I have only shared with a few people. It is not that I have kept this information secret, it is simply that I have not found the correct vehicle to pass on this information, until now. I have helped a few personal trainers get on their feet. I have done what I can to give them some advice and generally tried to be a good, community minded citizen by passing on information to help them. Whether they take up the opportunity to use this information is up to them. However, what I have passed on was limited because of our short time together. Some of the information I have detailed in this publication is unique to me and my previous training as a soldier, and to be honest, to those who have had the same or similar training. Very few in the health and wellness industry know the specific knowledge I have, due to my training. There are many, many trainers who are more successful than me, make more money and even have much better practices, but to be perfectly honest, if not a little immodest, I have been lucky to have been trained by some of the best people in this field.

You will learn how to handle large groups of people. Perhaps you are not setting out to do this, but if you are successful, eventually you may be placed in that position. You will also learn the pitfalls, and how to treat smaller groups of attendees. Both groups are important to your business, and although you may have all the necessary technical skills to teach a lesson, and identify the Latissimus Dorsi, your success as a personal and group trainer will largely be based on your skill at handling people, or if you prefer, "customer service". The same thing applies to personal training. I will discuss how you can be better as a personal trainer. Remember the personal part of personal trainer and don't expect miracles, because I don't profess that you will miraculously become brilliant. Of course, you still have to work very hard to be successful, but like a tradesman or apprentice starting out in the big world, you need to have a comprehensive toolkit. I will help you fill some of the gaps in your toolkit through this publication.

Do I have to be perfect?

You will learn it is much better to work towards perfection than to want to become a millionaire from health and wellness or the fitness industry. The harder you work, the better educated you become, the more you fine tune your skills, the more successful you become, and the income stream flows as a result. This fine tuning, of course, also applies to your business skills, which are extremely important.

The highs and lows

I discuss the highs and lows of personal and group training or the pros and cons and how I handle these situations. You have to develop your own skill set, but having a wealth of knowledge to choose from helps. I will provide some of this knowledge base in this book.

Dealing with the public demands a very disciplined and cheerful approach. It is not as easy as it may appear to be, and you have to be prepared for those people who are difficult to handle. I will give you some ideas on how you may handle these types of people.

Regulations

First Aid, rehabilitation and obligation or duty of care are other topics that we expand on in this book to give you an insight into how a working operation meets these regulations. It is great to have the theory, and it is an absolute must to keep up with the latest teachings and methods, but the practical, actual hands on dealing with these subjects and clients is important, and may be crucial to you and the ultimate success of your business.

I have not written in any depth about your business model. This is something that is entirely up to you and your advisers. It is personal, and everyone has a different model or expectation. I can give you a formula for fault correction that is universal. Businesses and how they are run depend on a number of factors and my only suggestion, which I make several times throughout this book, is to seek reputable, professional advice.

It is possible that a whole book could be made from every chapter in this publication, but time and space prevent me from going further. The information is detailed at times and general in other areas. What this book will do is stimulate your appetite, and get you thinking about the way in which you run your operation, whatever that may be. You will find some repetition in some areas of this book, and that is simply because some things need repeating. Perhaps by doing so, the points mentioned will be reinforced in your mind.

In the quest to be better, smarter, better informed, richer or just a much better all-round professional, this book will help. To most, it will provide additional information from which you can experiment and trial; at the very least it will give you an honest insight into the fitness industry from my own perspective, developed over more than 40 years, in various forms, in the physical fitness game. As I have been an independent manager of a medium-sized gymnasium, and a sole operator of a very successful business, I am sure you will find this book insightful, informative and of great use to you as a fitness provider. Good luck.

One of the things that has stayed with me from my school years is the way I learned to study. I am sure it came from my scribbled notes at school, when at night I would decipher the scribble and pick out the relevant parts to study and rewrite neatly. I got into the habit of highlighting what I thought were very important facts, statements or sentences. I still do this today when I read a reference book. I thought that to help you out, I would highlight those paragraphs, sentences or statements, in this book, that I believe you may want to highlight for yourself, or may be new to you, or assist you in some way.

1. Why do I work in the fitness industry?

I love what I do. I often think I must be the luckiest person in the world.

Well! It really is very simple. **I like being fit and healthy** and cannot imagine what it would be like now to be otherwise. I suppose this is only partly true, because I often say the motivation for me to remain relatively fit is the fact that I would not like to be trying to get fit. True, it really does not take anyone who is dedicated a long time to get back into shape, but I never want to be in that situation and hope I can keep well, fit and healthy for as long as possible. **Don't we all want that?**

I have been around fitness most of my life. As a little boy, I played many different sports, but mainly football (soccer). My father was very fit and instilled in us a sense of keeping the body healthy through exercise. Although football was my passion, I did represent my home town of Geraldton in Western Australia in amateur boxing, and up until a few years ago I still held the trophy from the 1967 WAABA Golden Gloves competition held in Perth, Western Australia. Yes, 1967, I was a 12-year-old. A strange combination perhaps, football and boxing, but as with most things in the formative years, children are influenced by what their parents do or wish for them. Strange as it may seem, my mother loved boxing and had relatives in Scotland who were reasonable boxers. My dad liked boxing as well, but loved football, so I did both for a number of years.

As a young man, I got caught up with the youth of my own age and started drinking, although I never really enjoyed drinking or the feeling I got from being drunk. We smoked too (although tobacco was my limit), and once again I took this up fairly late in life by comparison with my fellow apprentices.

Football remained a big part of my life and I was good enough to be selected, when I was 16, to play senior football. The boxing and the Geraldton PCYC became a distant memory, but I remain an admirer of boxing and actually use my previous training experience with my current aerobic boxing fitness classes. Incidentally, I remember well, my Uncle Reg (not really my uncle but a close family friend) giving me a boxing book when I was about 14 or 15 years of age, and among the high-lighted boxers was Cassius Clay, who won a Gold Medal at the 1960 Olympics. Cassius Clay, of course, went on to win the World Heavyweight Title three times as Muhammad Ali. In my opinion, he was the greatest boxer I have ever seen and one of the world's best sporting personalities.

Although as a youth I did some unhealthy things like smoking and drinking at times, generally we were very active. Smoking is no longer a part of my life and drinking is generally only socially now. As youths, our activity involved riding our bicycles to and from work or football training, and before this, we used to ride or walk to school. Exercise was part of daily life, and although my memory has become a little fuzzy with the passage of time, I can honestly only remember one overweight child in our class. I am pretty sure, based on my limited experience with children of school age now, that the ratio of slim to obese children would be very different. Anyway, you get the picture. I, like many in my era, did not have to go to gymnasiums or fitness classes to keep fit. Life and our daily routine, combined with organised sports, kept us all pretty lean and keen. Having said that, the PCYC was a club, and no one that I can recall ever called it a gym.

Nutrition was never something I considered as a younger man. My mother cooked what would now be considered a Paleo diet. Paleo (from the Palaeolithic era) is basically grass fed beef, fruit and vegetables with an absence or reduction of processed foods. The theory is based on the ancient cavemen and the hunter-gatherer period. Our family seldom had takeaway, and I was a teenager and driving a car when the first Kentucky Fried Chicken came to our town. Our diet was low in processed foods, very few soft drinks (mainly around Christmas time or family celebrations) and few sweets or lollies. Of course, we loved sweet foods, but by comparison with the abundance of desserts, confectionery, chocolates and all manner of lollies consumed today, we were not exposed to these much, because they were not as available.

There are many reasons why I work in this industry. Firstly, it is a very positive field to work in, and although there are some disappointments, generally the work is good, the people you work with are appreciative, and the scenery is fantastic. I am a mobile fitness provider and while I do use some indoor facilities, the great outdoors is a fantastic attraction for me. Yes, I did my stint in a gym, as a manager, and loved every minute of it, but my passion is training in the great outdoors. I seldom wore shoes as a kid, and only had a pair of shorts on when I was not at school. I was always tanned, and on more than one occasion it was thought that I was a young aboriginal boy. When I fought at the PCYC, I was given a pair of boxing trunks with "Choco" in big letters stitched down the side.

I suspect my years in the Army helped me understand

what we have here in Australia. I have also travelled overseas, and really believe that we are lucky here to have not only great weather, but some fantastic outdoor facilities, most of which are provided free by some level of government. This is really one thing I do appreciate. I cannot talk with any great authority about the facilities provided by any other country, but I believe we are very lucky in Australia. Our local authorities and councils provide every incentive, from free exercise sessions to great free local park equipment. There are few parks that you can go to in Australia that do not have some sort of play equipment for the children and fixed exercise stations for the youth and adults.

I like working for myself. Of course, I have worked for people for most my life, but I genuinely do enjoy being responsible for my own decisions and work ethic. I have had some employees and have found that, although they are good people, and more importantly from a business point of view, good workers, I generally like to do my own thing. Naturally, I get help when I can, and I do farm out work from time to time when it gets very busy for me, but most the time I do it all myself. I enjoy the challenge. I really believe the saying that a bad day in your own business is still better than a good day working for anyone else.

I like being fit and healthy. **What better way to help keep and maintain my fitness** than working in the industry. I have no doubt that some accountants feel the same about their jobs and carpenters, tradesmen and professional people like doctors, technicians and so on obviously enjoy what they do. I am just as sure that those who embrace what they do are very good, or working towards being very good, at their chosen profession or vocation.

There are many other reasons, from being stimulated by the company of a variety of different people and learning from their experiences and stories, to being excited by the challenge of providing appropriate exercises and even events. People who attend my sessions can expand their knowledge base and find, like I have, the joy and variety of physical and mental stimulation.

Although I did not expect this, and it did come as a little bit of a surprise, when you do personal training for people, they like to tell you things that are personal. I keep this information to myself, but like a taxi driver or barber, I think sometimes people like to tell you things that perhaps they cannot tell family or friends. It may be a way in which they offload or get things off their chest. Most of it is very pleasant and I love to hear how people interact with their family, children and grandchildren. Some of it is very informative and educational for me, and I learn a lot through these discussions. I suppose I am a sounding board as well as a personal trainer at times, although I do not give advice unless pressed and I try to keep it general. I think it is important to remember my area of expertise and not venture into areas I am not 100% familiar with or qualified in. It is very important for you to remember confidentiality of your client and the conversations you have. During the second world war, one of the common sayings was "Loose lips sink ships". It may not be as drastic as that, but keep your conversations private. Your reputation may suffer if you do not observe a client-in-confidence approach.

Just a word of warning here about relationships with your clients. I certainly have friends who do personal training with me, and some of them have become friends through personal training it's true. I always remember that our relationship is professional and I try very hard to keep the two separate. I do have very good friends who I take for personal training, and most of them became good friends via a long professional relationship. More is written about this later.

Though I have developed very good friendships with clients, we also have a mutual appreciation and respect for each other and our boundaries. As some of my very good clients have said, personal training is all about being personal and giving detailed attention to your client. Keep the relationship professional, and keep any friendship you have separated from the business side.

Group training presents a whole different set of challenges, and these keep me on my toes. I like to be able to make sure that my programs provide a physical workout for all who attend, and this is not always easy. Naturally, in any group you will find different body shapes and sizes, different ages, and men and women who have their own ideas about how to keep fit and what they want to do to achieve that. There is a whole chapter in the book on group training.

Experience is a wonderful thing, and I can tell you with all honesty I have made all the mistakes that anyone could think of, and more. Dealing with groups takes a particular skill, and not everybody has it. It can be developed and improved. No surprises here; it is exactly the same for any given occupation. I have come across the odd doctor or two who had no bedside manner whatsoever. They may have been very good general practitioners, but customer or client services have been sadly lacking. If your customer service skills are poor you will not only find it hard to keep clients, you will also struggle initially to find a client base suitable for sustaining your business. I will expand more on this later in the book. Just be aware that having the technical skills alone is not enough to make you competitive in what is becoming an increasingly popular industry.

The number one quality in any customer service business is that you must be a people person. I believe that

I am a people person and what I mean by this is that I genuinely like people and want to help them. If you work on this basis in most fields, from a customer service point of view, it is a great start. Do I get annoyed, am I accused of being grumpy, do people say, "He is having a bad day"? Yes Of course they do, but most people know and understand that I am trying to help them, and the odd off day is not desirable but inevitable in most occupations. So, trying to help people means that a manner that is acceptable in the least, but desirable at best, has to be developed.

There are days when some people seem to just want to test you and your patience, by not listening to instructions, doing the wrong exercise or blaming everything else except themselves. These days are sent to try us, and you will experience many of these if you work in the industry for long. The good days far outnumber any frustrations you may feel on days that test you. I consider myself lucky to have enjoyed all the jobs I have had in my life, although there were some days, in each job, that were challenging at some stage. I mention difficult people and some methods of dealing with them later in the book.

Once again, remember the good days are priceless. Clients tell you how much they loved the class. Feedback may come in a number of forms. You may get a glowing email or a Facebook review or comment. Some people will tell you directly, and it makes all the time and effort you have gone to worthwhile. You may even be fortunate enough to be given gifts, as well as being paid, by your loyal clients. I have been given fruit and vegetables, vouchers, alcohol, movie tickets, watches, heart rate monitors and even hands-free devices for my phone. People appreciate the effort that is put into keeping them as healthy as possible.

The time planning and rehearsing your class is well rewarded when the plan comes together and you get great feedback from your participants. You feel on top of the world when this happens and so you should. One of the best things to come out of consistently good sessions is that your clients will be so enthused that they will tell others, and this can only be good for you and your business. You cannot beat personal experience and positive word of mouth to help your business grow.

You feel good for so many reasons. A happy client is elated, and this feeling flows from them to their family and friends. Indirectly, you may have contributed to lifting the spirits of not just the person you have trained, but the entire family. Someone suffering depression, a lady who wants to get some shape back after having a child, a diabetic client, a cardiac rehabilitation patient, an attendee who has been told to get into shape before joining the armed forces, the list goes on.

Having said all the above, some of you are perhaps thinking of how you have the best job in the industry. You may be a personal trainer on a cruise ship, work in a family business or be a physical educational officer at a training establishment. Whatever dream job you have, like most of us in the industry you thrive doing it, and this makes a difference in how you perform. Those who are passionate about what they do in any field are easily recognisable by the energy and enthusiasm they display.

The hours I work suit me and my present lifestyle. Some people think I am a workaholic! At the time of writing this book I have just turned 61, but still like to work most days of the week. Currently, I work every day, but not every hour of every day. On my busy days, I do five sessions consisting of two group sessions and three individual programs. On the easiest day, I do only one group session. I like to keep busy and find that I have plenty of time for leisure and home-based activities working this way. It is a personal thing, and I do know a few group and personal trainers who work full-time but less hours. It is up to you and your circumstances. The main thing to remember is that the business is dynamic and will change on a regular basis. You need to keep up, and in some cases even be the catalyst that makes the changes.

I could go on a lot more about the benefits and how rewarding the job is or discuss more in depth some of the things that I will go into later in this book, but I think I have covered most of it, and I am sure you get the picture. You will no doubt discover many challenges and even some setbacks in your own career, but overall you are or will be working in a very exciting, dynamic and positive field. How well you do your job and the enthusiasm and energy you use, combined with your technical knowledge, can help to make the world a better place. Always keep that in mind. Good luck.

2. So you want to be a personal trainer?

Why not work in a field that keeps you fit, healthy and where you help other people to achieve the same?

Starting a chapter called "So you want to be a personal trainer?" may seem a little strange, as most of you who buy this book will be fully qualified or on the way to full qualification. I am sure you would be the first to agree there is a lot you do not get taught through the various teaching organisations, regardless of whether you did your course purely by correspondence, contact, part- or full-time. Even if you think you have learned it all in your learning institution, you will soon become aware, when you commence work, that you did not. You could not possibly be prepared for every situation that you will come across. Obviously, the main reason would be time restrictions, and in a group setting we know that not all of us learn well in classrooms.

Perhaps you are not currently qualified in our industry

regardless of the country you live in and intend to operate in but want to get more of an insight into the way the industry works. I have never believed it is possible to get too much information on any subject you are interested in and I am sure this book will help you in many ways to formulate your own opinion. It is not the be all and end all, but a lot of material is covered in these pages. Take your time reading this, take notes, highlight the areas you feel are important and keep it handy as a reference you can look back on anytime to reassure or remind you how to tread successfully through your career as a fitness provider.

I think many people see the fitness industry in a romantic way. I am not sure why this is the case. Perhaps a course that can be completed in less than two months (full-time) is attractive. Body image and the whole perfect body industry may have something to do with the attraction to the industry, **but don't be fooled!** To be good in this industry takes a lot of hard work, just as in any business or trade. As a manager of a gymnasium, I often had work experience students and young trainees attend our gym to gain real experience. They were attracted, in many cases, by the prospect of personal training and the thought of making a lot of money in an industry that is a very positive one, and one that promotes the perfect body image.

My emphasis is to basically give you what you need to

know as a group or personal trainer about the mechanics of running your own set-up and the actual working side. I do not want to get too involved with how you set up your business as an organisation. You may want to work full-time, part-time, in a gymnasium, by yourself in a sole operator style or as a company. This is entirely up to you, and although your various business arrangements may change depending on your circumstances, I will not be explaining in any depth the pros and cons of these arrangements. To be honest, I do not know enough about your circumstances or the regulations where you live, to give you worthwhile information, except to say get professional help. It is worth your while paying to get good advice from a person qualified in business management.

I have worked as a manager in a gym and have had two businesses with employees or partners. The experience I have gained from these, and throughout my life, leading up to managing and running my own operations, has taught me a great deal and given me the knowledge to not only run my own personal training and group training practice, but also to pass on some of this knowledge to you. I would not say, and could not possibly say, that I have no more to learn. I am still learning and enjoy learning more about this wonderful industry. I hope you do the same.

Seek knowledge. Listen to everyone's ideas about

your business, ask your parents, family and friends what they think, speak to people in the industry, seek professional advice, gather your information, and make informed decisions about your particular way of working in the industry. Make sure that if you are determined to succeed in this field, you do not get sidetracked. Speak only to people who can offer you good, sound advice. You know who they are, or you will soon after speaking to them. Most people can be as successful as they want to be if they adhere to some basic principles, so do not be deterred by negative or jealous people. For every positive person, you will find five negative people who want to tell you that it will never work. Listen to those you respect, and whose advice you trust, but do not be confused. Someone telling you the truth and pointing out pitfalls may not be negative, but simply forthright. My son reminds me from time to time that to have energy (like a battery) we need a negative and positive side, and this is true. You know what I mean. There are some people who, regardless of what you are talking about, have to put in their "two bob's worth", and more often than not it is the negative side of the story. Stay away from these people; they are energy thieves and dream destroyers.

Get some business skills. When I eventually left the military, I was as prepared as I possibly could be for business. I did several government-sanctioned courses on small business and basic marketing skills. These courses were just days long, not weeks, and they covered the basics of accounting, the marketing mix, and some money handling tips and taxation laws. I see no reason for anyone in our industry to pursue a degree in business management unless desired, but some formal business courses will stand you in good stead. Get some formal training relevant to the size of the business you are aiming for.

What are your costs? Regardless of where you work there will be costs. I know of some people who freelance and work only in public places and do so on an irregular basis. Because they are irregular and not working all the time in the same public place, they avoid site fees. But it will catch up with them eventually, and someone will complain. Perhaps it will be one of the regular PTs or trainers who do the right thing and pay the council for the site. It is better to be professional and do the right thing from the start, register your area, pay the fee and incorporate the cost into your business. I have had instructors tell me that they pay no costs for personal training because they do the training at the client's house. Unless they walk there, they have to incorporate transport into the cost of the session. Even sessions at your own house or studio incur costs for things such as electricity, water, equipment, repairs and cleaning. Nothing is free, and there is a cost to you, so make sure you consider this when planning your sessions and costing your effort and expertise. Your time is important, and you need to cost this also. Just because you have not spent any money does not mean it is free. Time and expertise should be considered and costed. **Check out the costs associated with starting up a business in your area, including insurances, permits, council approval and so on.**

What will you charge? It is not my business nor my intention to tell you what to charge for your services, but I do want to let you in on some advice. Don't be fooled by those people who tell you that you can charge big because you now have your Certificate IV or Diploma and that the cost of you studying can be borne by your clients; this is rubbish. You obtain more qualifications initially because you want to be better at what you do. When you are good at what you do, then the money becomes a less important factor because people will pay for good services and good operators. I know of people who have minimum qualifications and they have a good income because they are good at what they do. Qualifications do not give you an automatic license to think that you can charge people more money.

Look at the market. Since I have been doing group training, I do not think the standard price of $10 per person per session has moved much. Yes, of course, some people charge $15 a session, some even $5 a session, but in both instances, you need to look at what is being provided. I have some concerns about paying too much, and similar concerns about not paying enough. Some operators work on payment plans per week and other types of deals. The market generally will determine what a fair price is and the rest is up to you. Before you start your operation, you need to address your expectations. Do you want five people at $15 each or 15 at $10 per person?

Consider this: A 20-year-old who has recently qualified, and now has a Certificate IV in personal training, decides to charge $15 a head for their group training program. Operating nearby is a trainer who has been in the market for a few years more than our recently qualified Certificate IV trainer, and they provide group training for $10 per session. The fee charged is seen as disproportionate to experience. It may not be the case, but the perception certainly will be that it is.

What about PT? As I write this, I am aware that some gyms in my area in greater Brisbane allow their PTs to charge whatever they want. Obviously, the market will settle on what is fair and reasonable, but many of the gyms have a business model that ensures they get rent from the instructor, so the personal trainer has to set their price in a range that ensures they can pay the rent before any money is made. Although I have never worked in a gym that works like this, I did have one of my staff leave our employment for a large gym, to work on a rental basis. The staff member was working for me on wages and left to work at a much larger gym that did not pay wages but worked on a contract system with instructors, where rent was paid. The theory was that a good PT could make a lot of money. Unfortunately, the reality was different. The gym already had a number of PTs, and eventually my ex-employee moved on to a more successful business model.

Contract work is good provided you can make enough money to pay your way, and like any business, the better you are, the more popular you become. A good PT contracted to a gym may be charging a high price for their services, and if people are happy with this service, they will pay that amount. The market sets its own level.

If you work for yourself, then you simply need to set a price that the client is happy to pay, and you are happy with, as fee for service. A set price is good as a basis to work from, but travel, multiple sessions and location all come into the mix, and you need to bring these factors into your calculations.

Note: Ask this question to those personal trainers who claim to be charging excessive amounts of

money per personal training session: "How many clients at this rate do you have?" Once again, the bottom line is that you should do your research and charge fairly and competitively. I have come across many very positive young trainers and in discussions with them they have told me that they value their own time and will charge a premium. I admire their pluck, but the value you place on yourself may not be the same value that a client is prepared to pay. Keep this in mind.

One size does not fit all. This is so true in group training and personal training. The reason some people attend your sessions is that they want the interaction of a person helping them, correcting them, and generally making them healthier and fitter. Plus, it is your energy that motivates them. They cannot get this from a computer program that tells them what to do with a few diagrams, and videos with instructions on what to eat, and how many calories to consume; that is why they like what you do. Naturally, there is a market for the computer program, but I am not writing about this. So, firstly, understand that we all have different needs, we work differently, have different capabilities and injuries and may not be able to do a burpee six ways, so flexibility and compassion is a great asset to have in your personal training and group training locker. The way you develop this is by practice, rehearsal and by increasing your knowledge base. Be like a sponge and take in everything you can from the industry.

Practice means you actually enact what you are going to do, and in so doing you learn, by practice, what works, what doesn't, and what seemed to be easy in the lesson plan you wrote up but is in fact a little more difficult. While you know this and have been taught this, it has been my experience that some do not practice much, if at all, after qualification. Practicing prevents any unforeseen event disrupting your session. It keeps you sharp!

Rehearsals are different from practice because you can practice anywhere, but a rehearsal should be done in the same location as your session. Practice can be a section of your session, and be done in the car, in the bathroom or anywhere really as you practice your method of delivery. A rehearsal should be in the exact location where you intend facilitating so you can work your space, see the area you are going to work in, and physically do a set-up of the equipment and apparatus. It is too late when you arrive for your session early only to find that the space you need is not available, simply because you did not check out the site and do a rehearsal. Keep in mind, however, that from time to time you may have to do an unrehearsed session in a completely new area. This should be the exception and not the rule.

On-site rehearsals should be done, if possible, at

the same time you intend doing your session, so that factors like the light, position of the sun, noise and public distractions are taken into consideration and adjustments made, if any, during the rehearsal.

Your knowledge base can be improved in a number of ways, and not simply by time spent in the job. Firstly, do some research, ask colleagues, observe other fitness providers, read about what the latest trends, methods and systems being used are, and most importantly be open to everything. I like to observe other operators, and I often get great ideas just by observing them. It is true that sometimes you see behaviours that are undesirable or not ideal, but this is good too because you can make a mental note not to use these methods of instruction. You gain experience by watching those who are very good at their craft and sometimes those who are not so good.

Competition is good. A mate of mine who runs a very successful business and meets a lot of people keeps telling me that everyone he meets is a personal trainer. There is a fair bit of exaggeration here, but the point is there are a lot of personal trainers in the market. I am only basing this on my experience, but I do believe that many qualified personal and group trainers work in other fields, simply because it is not as easy to set up a business as you may think. Let's face it: getting a fitness qualification does not take years, and some may see it as a means to get a quick qualification and start their own business. Good luck, I say, but be aware that competition is good; it can, and will, make your job more challenging.

An instance where competition can be a really good thing is that you can choose to set your business up the same as everyone else, competing for the same market, or you can seek out your own niche in the market to entice clients to your new business. Young mums often cannot make early morning sessions and may prefer to work out between the hours of 9am–11pm. Working people might prefer to get their exercise session out of the way early. Children need sessions after school hours, shift workers are only available at certain times and so on. Work out your demographic and cater to it; this is my suggestion. Once again, you should do your research and spend some time looking at the market share you desire. A younger trainer I now know quite well was watching me work my group for nearly the entire session and after we had finished, she approached me. She introduced herself and mentioned she was looking at starting up a regular class in the area I was using but at a different time. This lady then asked me if I minded answering some questions she had and I said no problems. She was doing her research, and I left the area thinking what a switched-on trainer she was. The interview with me was part of her homework. Since that time, this lady has become one of the very good operators in our area, and I have even handed over some classes to her.

Starting out can be soul destroying, but don't give up. Some people thrive on selling and being upfront, and have no problem pushing themselves or their product. Some people are not good at doing this. Last week one of my personal training competitors came and chatted to me about his business. After a few years, he decided to fold and work for someone else. He explained to me that while he loved his work, he did not have any real business skills. He was very honest, and I admire this in him. Very few of us have the whole package, but you need to be able to sell yourself and your programs, because no one else will do it for you. Keeping this in mind, be realistic about how long it may take you to get your business going. Some trainers prefer to work part-time, on weekends or when the work presents itself. Others work part-time, intending to gradually secure enough work to go full-time in the industry. Don't be deterred. If your dream is to be the next Michelle Bridges or Commando, then get out and start working. Be smart, do your homework, be good at what you do, and work at it daily and you will get your breakthrough. Your name may not end up in lights, and you may not get your own TV show, but you can be successful. **Keep at it!**

Your summer and winter group. You will quickly learn that your group training numbers will fall in winter and pick up in summer, regardless of whether you have wet weather facilities or not. It was true in the gym that I managed, and it is true in my mobile outdoor business.

In Australia, we do get some extremes of temperature and wild weather. That is true. But if I use my own business as an example, I can only count a handful of instances where extreme, inclement weather caused me to cancel any of my sessions. The reason for the cancellations, in every instance, was based on safety. It can be dangerous during our summer storms for people to travel to the session, and it is better to cancel rather than allow people to risk their own safety to attend PT or group training. **One of the very well respected and popular yoga teachers I know who operates in the same area as us, Monica Batiste, posted a comment on Facebook about us after she conducted a yoga session with only four people attending. Monica said, "I take my hat off to Tom's Law, because he has seasoned his team to be out in all kinds of weather. Two participants on this morning are Tom's Law fans too. I really don't see why we can't stay on the beach all winter."**

Human nature dictates that during the cooler months, people are inclined to drop off and return in summer. Ask anyone who has worked in this field for a while, and they will tell you that it is important not to get concerned when your numbers drop in winter, as generally they will pick up again when the weather starts getting warmer. You and I know that the summer body is generally made in the cooler months as well as the warmer ones, and those who exercise should strive for consistency and exercise all year round, but in reality, it does not happen. Just be aware of it, and continue to keep contact with all your clients. Some will even tell you up front that they will be taking some time off exercise in winter, only to return in summer. I must admit that many of our clients keep exercising in the outdoors in winter because I do. If the instructor cannot handle inclement weather, it will naturally follow that the clients will not attend.

It is a numbers game. When you start out in this business, most of you will find the hardest thing is to convince people to come and exercise with you. Personal training or group training, regardless of where you are conducting your business, requires clients, and getting those clients, for many people, is one of the hardest things to do. We discuss how you may attract clients a bit more in chapters 8 and 9, but the important thing is to build as large a client base as possible for the following reasons. If you have worked hard and now have a group of 10 people coming a few times a week, and four or five people doing PT with you, then that is a good start. However, keep in mind that people go on holidays, get sick, injured, have to work back, find money tight at times, or stay away because of the weather. Whatever the reason, your 10 clients may only equate to two or three turning up. **My client database is over 1,000, but I have had two sessions over the years where we had as few as two turn up for a class. So, keep in mind that while you enjoy small group training, and only a few PT clients, you need to have a larger base to support that smaller-sized group turning up. Once again, the business side of the fitness industry is very important.**

Don't stop learning. Of course, in Australia it is mandatory to provide evidence of professional development in our industry. Annually, we are required to gain Professional Development Points (PDPs) or Continuing Education Credits (CECs). This is a great idea and encourages us to ensure that we continue to strive to be abreast of the latest developments in the industry. Naturally, this subject (PDPs, CECs) relates to all in the industry in Australia, but it is worth mentioning in this book as it is often seen as an inconvenience rather than an opportunity. My advice is to keep across all developments in the industry regardless of your direct involvement or not. As an example, I am aware of the popularity and benefits of Zumba to the physical fitness community, but I personally do not teach it. My point is that although your own personal preference may be CrossFit, for example, you should not close yourself off to other practices or disciplines in the fitness industry. All disciplines have an audience and fulfil a purpose.

Our industry, like many others, is very dynamic. The science of physical movement and anatomy is very exciting and always in the media spotlight. Keep up with the latest trends, read, study and always remain a student of your trade. It will stand you in good stead.

3. Don't search for wealth; strive to be better; wealth may follow

"It doesn't matter who you are, how old you are or how much money you have, many of us get to a stage in life where we start to think about our longevity and health. For some, unfortunately, it may come too late. Don't regret not looking after your body and your well-being and make a start now. Education programs around the world are advising us through all forms of media to start looking after ourselves. Good health is not only beneficial individually, but it also reduces the cost to government-funded health care. You may be surprised at the results from some regular activity, and the benefits are too numerous to mention. You owe it to yourself and your family to be the best you can be, and that certainly includes your health. Life is movement, keep moving."

I wrote the above for a Facebook post a while ago, and I believe it to be true. You may have a lot of money, but health is the real wealth, and this is great for anyone in the fitness industry because we are always going to have plenty of raw material to work with. Of course, there is competition, but one of the main considerations when going into any business is the target market. According to a Suncorp Bank study, Australians currently spend more than $8.5 billion each year in gym memberships, sports equipment and the latest fitness fads. This equates to approximately $2,340 per household. Naturally, we would expect this trend and numbers to increase, not fall. The point I am making is that there is plenty of room for you, if you are good at what you do, and good at running a business.

I hear from some in our industry how they make a lot of money via personal training. Well, it has been my experience that the people who make the money are those who tell you **how** to make money in the industry. Okay, you may be the next Les Mills, Lorna Jane or Commando, but really, only a few successful people make their money in television, clothing or exercise program distribution and licensing. This does not mean that you cannot make a decent living out of doing personal training or group training, but think about it for a few minutes, and tell me five people you know who have become millionaires through personal and group training. Even if you use the three people I have already mentioned (assuming they are all millionaires), you will struggle to name five. You will find it much easier to name five very rich media and mining personalities.

While researching for this book, and particularly this chapter, I spoke to many operating in the health and wellness field, and most agree that there is a fair bit of competition around, though the market, as stated above, is enormous. This being the case, most clear minded people would do their research when selecting a person to train with, be it in a group or personal training context. To be competitive, you not only have to be good at what you do, but your price range must be in the ballpark with most other facilitators. Although you may hear differently, and I certainly have, I have not met anyone who is not concerned about how much they are charged for PT or group training.

If we assume that generally, among the run of the mill group and personal training facilitators, there is not much variation in price, then other considerations for a potential client would be venue, location, experience, qualifications and how good you are in your field. Potential clients may not do as much research into their personal training or group trainer provider as they might when purchasing a car or house, but seldom do they throw themselves into a program without firstly doing some research. **From my time in the industry, I can tell you that most people who attend my sessions come to me via a word of mouth recommendation.**

45

Advertising is good, but can be expensive. So, unless you have a lot of money to spend, you need to rely on other sources of promotion. I find word of mouth is by far the most effective and certainly the cheapest form of advertising. From my research with other instructors, word of mouth is also a big part of their success.

So, back to my chapter heading. Don't search for wealth. Strive to be better; wealth may follow. Those who seek money at the expense of being a good operator in their field may make money initially, but in the long run, they will be found out and clients will vote with their feet. Don't get me wrong. If you are not in business to make money, then you should not start one. I have no issue with any business making a healthy profit, but what can happen, and unfortunately does happen, not just in our industry but others, is that some people seek only wealth and then other areas of the business suffer. Remember that people are not stupid, and they will see through the fact that you are solely focused on making money.

My advice to you is this. Be as good as you can be at your trade, work hard, keep updated, go on courses and learn the art of effective communication. Be considerate to your clients and give them good advice. If you don't know the answer to their questions, refer them to someone who does. I don't mean you have to pamper your clients, as they seldom want this, but they do need a considered and individual approach to their needs. Don't try and make out that you know everything; develop associations with health-related experts and refer your clients to them if necessary.

It really gets down to being genuine about how you go about your business. Your clients pay for a service, and you need to provide that service. Call it value for money if you like. In my business, I certainly upsell. As with other similar organisations, we sell caps, T-shirts, singlets and hoodies in winter. There is nothing wrong with this, and you can supplement your income by making a profit on these items, and other services, but it must be seen to be good value for money. Good value for money means that you know your core business and charge accordingly. It means that you keep abreast of the latest developments, and professional development, and that you become successful by running a credible organisation where your combination of service and professionalism make you an attractive proposition for potential clients.

To those in the industry, old or new, who think that the health and fitness game is a vehicle to make a lot of money, I offer them good luck. Many before you have tried, and a few, to be honest, have succeeded. Those who have succeeded in a big way have no doubt worked hard with great passion and professionalism, a fantastic business plan and vision! The other thing they would all have is a burning desire to be as good as they possibly could. You may not be the next celebrity fitness host of "The Biggest Loser", or have the fame and fortune of Michelle Bridges, but by being as good as you possibly can you are giving yourself every chance of running a successful business. **Be good at what you do and work at it; the money will naturally follow.**

Later in this book, I explain how my business works and how I make my money as a personal trainer and group trainer. You need to find something that works for you. It may be the traditional model or something that you have designed.

Naturally, a lot of time spent in business training revolves around making a profit. Of course, the number one reason we are in business is to make a profit, and if you don't want to do that then don't go into business. Your ability to make money is directly related to providing the best client services you can, combined with a good business plan, and combined with the ability to implement it.

I have mentioned an instructor who I know quite well, who is a terrific trainer and has a good following, but by his own admission is no good at business so he has returned to working for someone else. Not everyone is suited to running their own business, but once again if you are very good at what you do, and highly sought after, many rewards will follow, including financial benefits.

This is an exciting field to be working in, and my hope is that many of you reading this are starting out in the fitness game. I am still learning and feel motivated and excited about my business and the area in which I work. The health and wellness field is one that will not fade away like some businesses that have become redundant, such as bookshops and video stores. Many studies have confirmed what a lot of us already know: that the health and wellness field will continue to grow, and I honestly believe that we will soon see a major shift in government policy and subsidies to encourage a healthier population. Currently, we are spending millions of dollars in taxpayers' money, healing those suffering diabetes, obesity, heart disease, and poor health and nutrition. I believe that we need to stop placing the ambulance at the bottom of the cliff, and start focusing on prevention. Prevention is the best cure.

Lastly, the title of this chapter **"Don't search for wealth. Strive to be better; wealth may follow"**, is worth thinking about again. Of course, you want to make money, as I have already mentioned. Think about any business you may be involved in or want to start. It would be foolish to start a business without having a good general knowledge of most, if not all, aspects of the business. The only reason the title says "wealth may follow" instead of "wealth will follow" is because it is up to you and what you want to do with your business. I know of several businesses that are very successful but do not want to be much bigger. If you want to conquer the world with your particular fitness regime and be the next big thing, make sure that you occasionally read this chapter again, and strive to be better. Good luck!

4. *Do as I do and do as I say*

Every day I try to learn a bit more about this industry. I might observe another instructor, read a book or go online to fine tune my knowledge. I also practice every day so that I can keep my fitness skills as finely tuned as possible. It is great to see a trainer in control of his body and his clients. The chapter title comes from a saying like one my dad always used, except he told us to "do as I tell you, not do as I do".

Each day at my programs, like thousands of people like me in our industry, I give demonstrations and explanations of the exercise we are about to undertake. It is a given that good demonstrations must be performed. It is not enough for you to simply tell a group of people to do 50 push-ups and leave it at that, without a full explanation and demonstration. The exception to this may be when the group of people who you are instructing have been with you for a while and understand the exercise and the technique. The way you do this is important.

Explanations, demonstrations, and even simple demonstrations of part of an exercise, may have to be performed in stages. An example of this might be a burpee. A complete demonstration of the burpee, followed by the burpee in stages and an explanation, may have to be given to those who are new to this exercise. I must admit that even the experienced attendees at my group and personal training still require a complete demonstration of certain exercises every time we do them.

Don't fall into the trap of assuming that everyone knows the exercise you have suggested. I have, and need to remind myself! There is a tendency for those of us in the field to assume that everybody knows all the exercises, or most of them. There are many people out there who need a simple demonstration of the most common exercises, so always make sure your group is well and truly aware of what you mean, and the way in which you want it performed.

Just a note here to keep in mind. If you have an attendee who also goes to the gym or another trainer, then they may do the exercise you want them to do in a slightly different way. Just be aware and explain the differences. I generally tell people who do the exercises differently to what I expect, or have different names for the exercises, that this is the way we do it. There is no wrong way (poor and dangerous form excepted), only different.

I would like a dollar for every time a new person came to our exercise group session and was shown how we do our sit-ups and crunches, for example. There are often many different ways in which similar exercises are executed, so just ensure you demonstrate and explain how **you** want them done. Hand in hand with this is the fact that many exercises have different names like plank, bridge or arch. All these are names for the same exercise. In Australia, we do star jumps, but Americans call them jumping jacks.

A word of warning. Demonstrations need to be done correctly or as you require them to be done. As an instructor, it is assumed that you would do near perfect demonstrations but, unfortunately, this is not always the case. I have seen experienced fitness providers in and around where I work, and I have to say that not all demonstrations are great. I don't mean the odd slip or bad form that can happen to any of us; what I am talking about is poor demonstrations to clients that invariably lead to the client performing badly executed exercises. If you are not sure how to do the exercise you are going to demonstrate, then make sure you get plenty of practice well before your scheduled session. Get some help to check your form also. If you continue to have difficulty executing a particular exercise, then perhaps you should shelve it and not use it until you can demonstrate it correctly. If you cannot do the exercise correctly, then how can you expect your client to do it correctly?

Bad form, posture or body shape, whatever you want to call it, consistently demonstrated by a qualified person in the fitness industry, will not be particularly inspiring to those who you are trying to instruct in the correct methods. Believe it or not I have seen this happen. Luckily it does not happen often, but it does happen. Your credibility as a facilitator will certainly diminish if this practice continues, and your business may be adversely affected. I encourage all our clients to continually correct theirs and others' form if it is not being executed correctly. This is done in an encouraging way, and is not in any way a negative thing. At all my classes, I ask the student to assess my demonstrations to ensure that the best possible demonstration is being delivered.

How you conduct your classes has a real bearing on your popularity and subsequently your business. If you are employed by someone, then it may affect your employer's business and this will affect you in some way, I am sure.

A successful business depends on a number of factors. One that is very close to my heart is the example you set as an instructor, your style of instruction and interaction with your clients. **Your style is something you develop that probably has a lot to do**

with your personality, character and experience base. Often, this is the difference between being a run of the mill operator or very successful. Let's face it, all of us have done nationally accredited courses that basically teach the same thing, so one of the main points of difference is how we deliver the training we have received, and our interaction with our clients. You may find that some people are not particularly keen on your style or manner or any other trait that you may have. Don't be discouraged unless the number gets to epidemic proportions. You cannot be everything to everyone.

Some trainers present in a way that I call Stand and Deliver. This is exactly what it says: they run their programs by simply dictating what the client is to do and watching them do it. They may have a timer in their hands, or as seems to be the modern trend, a phone from which they take their notes and timing. One operator I observed the other day had his hands in his pockets while issuing orders. These types of trainers are not unlike the early morning trainers you may see on the horse racetrack. The trainers are rugged up against the cold, and have a stopwatch in hand timing their horseflesh on the track. Just look around: it happens too often. Not particularly inspiring!

One image I will never forget is of a group of people performing on the beach near where I live. The group was quite large and there were two instructors. I could tell they were in charge because they were the only two people standing upright, while their clients were doing push-ups and other exercises in the sand. The two instructors had jackets on, printed with "Coach" on the back. You may have now worked out what type of fitness group they were. Regardless, I have seen funny things from all fitness types. The really disappointing thing about these coaches was that they both had takeaway coffees in their hands and were sipping them between barking out instructions. I remember thinking two things at the time. Firstly, the group and coaches were very fit and muscular and were working hard, and that was impressive. Secondly, I thought to myself that the coaches may be very good at their job, but drinking coffee, standing upright with jackets on, and barking orders to their clients was not my idea of inspirational leadership by example. Not a professional look! The Army had a very unique way of dealing with people like this, and while the pressure and intensity in military training may be more extreme than civilian boot camps, some of the principles remain the same.

Another instructor I observed turned up in thongs one day. His group wore shoes, and understandably so, but the sight of an instructor in a public place in thongs is not only unprofessional, it reflects badly on that particular instructor, the industry and, more importantly, on that instructor's business. That's not even to mention the health and safety aspect. Now, there may be reasons for wearing thongs, perhaps a foot injury or a specific medical requirement prevented a shoe from being fitted. In this case, it can be excused, but I would rather hand over my class to someone on a temporary basis until my injury was healed sufficiently to wear a shoe again. Can you imagine any workplace, with the possible exception of beach lifesaving, where thongs are considered appropriate dress?

Below is my method. It is not unique to me. I used it for many years in the Army, and I must admit it was the military that taught me how to present in the way that they wanted. I still use these methods every day, the formula is easy to follow, and once you know it you use it constantly. It makes for a more productive class when the passage of information is effective. The reason these methods are good is that the military has developed these systems for the masses. In a group situation, there is no time for individual instruction, except when dealing with specific more detailed instructions. These systems are tried and tested, and work for most people. Civil institutions have adopted similar methodologies over the years.

Demonstrate – Explain – Practice. (DEP) Firstly, give a good demonstration, followed by a detailed explanation, then as a group, practice. Now, I have seen similar methods in use but believe that this method is simple, easy to understand and, importantly, easy to assimilate. The client sees you demonstrate, you then explain what you have done, followed by the client practicing. Many of you may have used similar or even the exact method, however, it is important that you do not vary this at all. An example of trying to shortcut or vary the DEP method is where the instructor tries to demonstrate and explain at the same time. There is a time and place for this, but this method is one of the easiest to learn and perform. I use this method on a daily basis.

Demonstrate – Demonstrate – Explain – Practice. (DDEP) A more detailed demonstration is given, followed by a demonstration of a part of the exercise, with an explanation and practice to follow. An example of this is the "clean and jerk". A demonstration of the full movement is given, followed by a demonstration of the "clean" then practice the "clean". The same process would be undertaken for the "jerk". After completing a practice of all the segments, a practice of the full movement would take place. This method is used where you need to pass on more information, and the movements are not simple. Another exercise I use this for, particularly for newer clients, is the burpee. I will give a full demonstration of the entire movement, followed by an explanation of the first part of the burpee, then get the client to practice. Next I would move onto the second part of the movement and so on. I use this method when taking people over obstacle courses. I demonstrate the method of execution over the obstacle, then break it down into sections, demonstrating and explaining each movement. I particularly choose to use this method with personal training. It is a good system to use when teaching more complex movements, or where the client or clients are relatively new to exercise.

Explain – Practice. (EP) This is the simplest method and the one I use most, particularly with people who are regulars and know the exercises well. An example would be where I instruct the group to start performing crunches. All that is required is to tell them what to perform and they commence. Another example would be "on go, start doing star jumps or jumping jacks". You could also use "I want you to run up this set of stairs to the top and back down to the bottom five times – ready, go". You have simply explained what to do, and the group will commence when you give them the instruction. Not rocket science, I agree, but a consistent method of passing on information with a brevity of words.

Demonstrate and Practice. (DP) This method is particularly good where the group or individual has been exercising for some time, and a demonstration may be academic, but lets the person or group know the way that you want the exercise done. Demonstrate the exercise and get the client to practice. Little or no explanation is required, and the client can start the exercise quickly and not be hindered by any lengthy explanation.

Rules or guidelines are flexible, as are my guidelines for demonstrations and practice, but you should be conscious of attempting to demonstrate and explain at the same time. There are some instances, without doubt, where you need to stop midstream and explain what you are doing. But unless you are very adept at this skill, as some are, you should avoid it and the possibility of the confusion which may cause you to lose your way or at the very least lose some confidence.

Teaching, demonstrating and explanations are often the hardest things for students to become adept at. When we start to formalise methods of instruction it can appear daunting, and there is no doubt that when most of us are placed in front of a crowd we can be intimidated. The beauty of using a system is that you do not have to develop your own, and once you have mastered any method it automatically becomes part of your presentations. Systems prevent chaos, confusion and uncertainty for the instructor. A clear, concise and well-communicated message with good demonstrations is the basis of your skills as a presenter, facilitator and instructor. Make sure you pay enough attention to practicing your presentation, demonstration and explanation skills. **Note: I have been in the industry for long enough to know and remember the pitfalls and failures that I and others have had. One of the reasons for writing this book is to inform those who are setting out in the industry of these, and to pass on my experience.** I consider myself to be a reasonable communicator, but even in my groups, which can be over 40 people, some clients do not always understand my explanations. I see this as my failure to communicate properly, not their problem. Most of us comprehend differently and, as trainers, we need to understand that not everybody gets it at the same time or by the same method.

I recall many times when I worked in a gym I would see people clearly doing the wrong exercise or an exercise incorrectly. When I approached them to correct what they were doing, many would tell me that they did not completely understand what was demonstrated and explained to them on induction, or when their program was presented to them. Although you may think, initially, that this is the client's fault, it is not. The problem is with the person conducting the program. Often, we as trainers can take a client for granted, and a gym orientation may be rushed. Remember the client may not be back at the gym for a few more days and may forget the program or sections of it. Some gym members are too embarrassed to ask, and just soldier on doing the wrong thing. We averted this in the gym by making sure that the client was shown their program again when they came to the gym a second time. Not every new client needed this reinforcement. You will find, in most gyms, a number of clients who are not only competent at what they do, but they are also students of health and wellness, and therefore great exponents of a variety of exercises.

The client needs to feel comfortable and be able to say, "Can you demonstrate that again please?" or "Can you show me that again and explain what muscle group I am working here please?". The only way a client will feel happy to do this is if you can convey to them your desire to help them. **Keep in mind that, as the trainer, you are the expert in this field, and don't take for granted that everybody knows what a lat pulldown is.** In a survey I did many years ago when I managed a gym, a lot of people wrote how even though gym staff may be very approachable and helpful, they still feel silly asking for advice or another demonstration on how to use equipment or how to perform a specific exercise. Keep in mind that some people have just joined your gym or exercise program for the very first time, and you may need to spend more time with these clients.

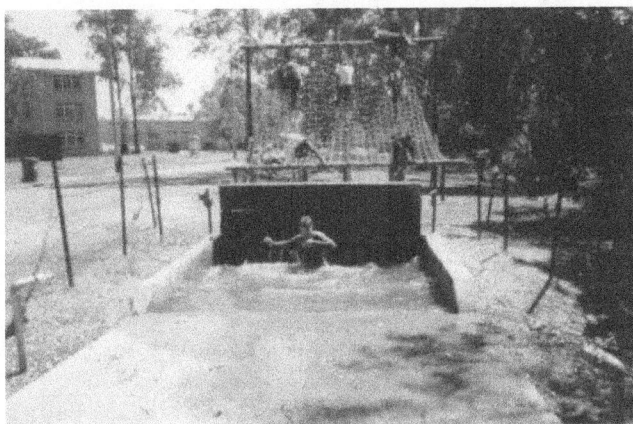

1. Water obstacle at a confidence course.

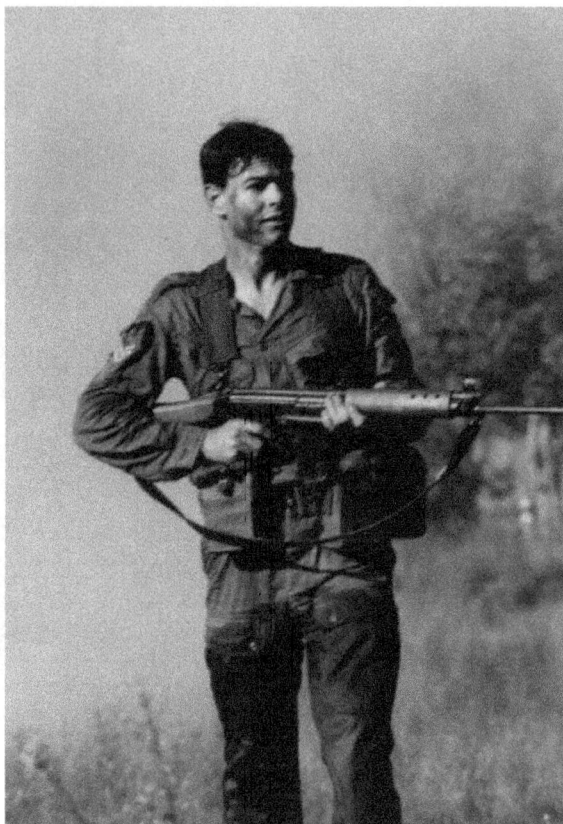

2. Sergeant Law: at the Australian Army's First Recruit Training Battalion in my role as a Drill Instructor, 1985.

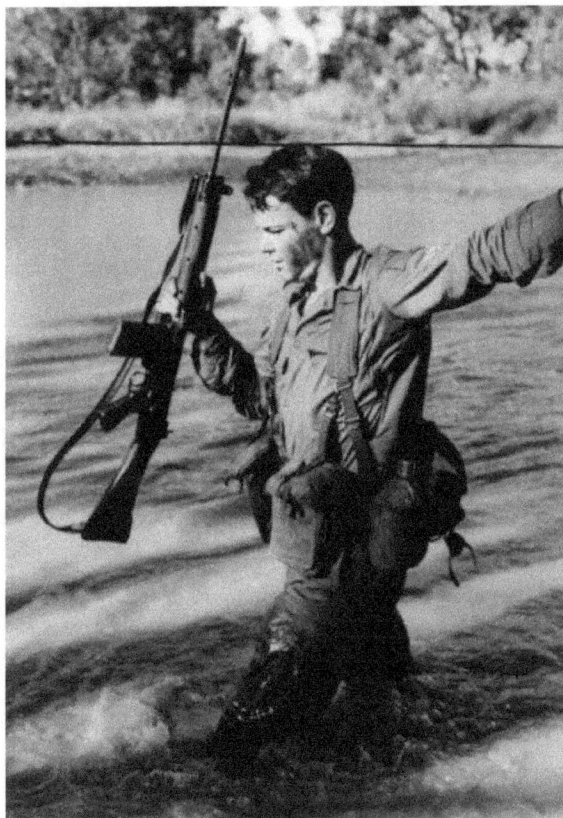

3. Battle inoculation training.

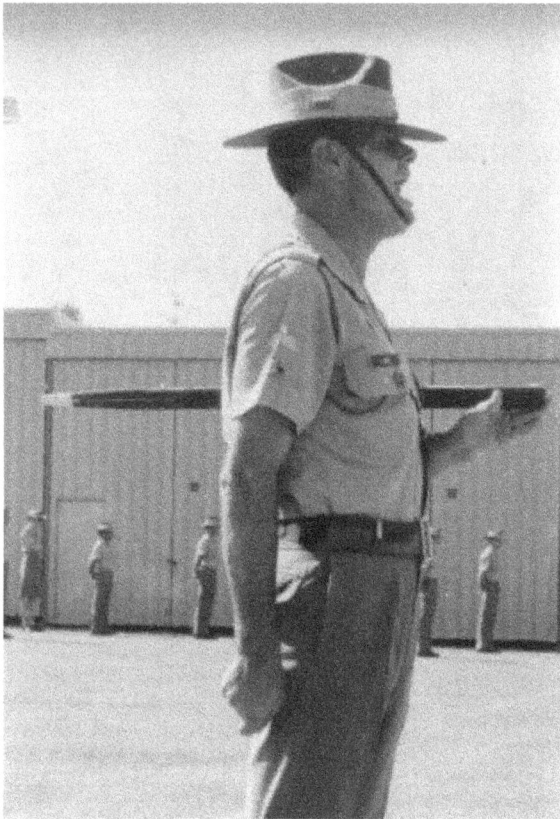

4. Regimental Sergeant Major Law at the
1st Signal Regiment.

5. *Fault correction, fault correction, fault correction*

From my observations over many years I would say that a lack of good, positive fault correction by the trainer is one area that can be improved dramatically.

If you asked any person who attends my group training sessions, I believe most would tell you that I am a stickler for good posture and form. To ensure your charges achieve this, you have to constantly give feedback and correct faults. Most people who attend your session will have as one of their objectives a desire to be able to do the exercises you prescribe correctly. Keep that in mind and remind yourself of that regularly.

The golfer Gary Player is fond of the saying, **"The harder I practice, the luckier I get"**. I love that saying because it is like one I use all the time: **"The harder I practice proper form, the better I become at it"**. I like to tell all who attend my group or personal training that coming to exercise in any capacity is great. Once you have made the decision to do it, then the next thing you should want is do it as best you can. **In our game, we call it form.**

I think there are three main aspects of fault correction, and while you may know what they are, sometimes we need to remind ourselves of their importance. (There are many more aspects of fault correction, but these my main ones.)

The first element of fault correction is good demonstrations. Imagine, as an instructor, how your credibility would take a dive if you gave poor demonstrations. How much worse would it be if, having demonstrated a particular exercise or move very badly, you then insisted that your clients do it properly? You need to practice good demonstrations and even get someone to check out your form. There is nothing wrong with having someone who you can trust coach you and make sure your form is good. It is something we should never forget and even now, when I turn up for a session and have the area set up, I go through some rehearsals and check my form before the session commences. Having no mirrors may be the only disadvantage associated with working in the great outdoors. Most gyms have plenty of large mirrors strategically located, where gym members can check out their exercise posture at any time.

There will be times when you are not 100% well, and while, in an ideal world, you would take some time off and get a replacement, it is not always possible. In these situations, it is perfectly acceptable for you to use a participant as an example, and get them to demonstrate the position or exercise.

A word of caution here. Make sure that the person you have selected is happy to be the training aid, check that their form is good, and make sure you both get a chance to do a rehearsal at least once. This technique can be used not only when you as the instructor are injured or incapacitated, but also when the person you select is very good at a particular exercise or movement. There are many people in my classes who are not only as good, but better than me at particular movements and exercises, and if they agree it is a great option to ask them to demonstrate. Often the client will enjoy the recognition as well.

Secondly, you have to develop a method of fault correction that doesn't embarrass or belittle your clients. There will be some people, who, regardless of how many times you correct their posture or positioning, will seldom adopt the perfect form. You need to be aware that this person still requires your attention but not exclusively or to the detriment of the other attendees. Make sure that you are not singling out a particular person, and if they are continual offenders, then perhaps you can have a word to them after the session or privately at a more convenient time. Work on fault-correcting techniques and practice what you are going to say. **"Lower your backside slightly, Julie." "Spread your feet to approximately shoulder width, John." These are just two examples of some fairly gentle but direct fault correction. You will note that there is no need to touch the client. This is very important.** We will mention physical contact later. I always try to inject some humour into the situation, particularly if the session is going to be tough. Humour should be natural and not forced. Sarcasm or humour that offends your clients is unprofessional. Your reputation will be damaged if you embarrass or belittle clients, even if it is disguised as humour. I must admit that this is one area that I believe a lot of younger people in the industry are very good at. They seem to be able to gently correct without upsetting or disappointing their clients.

My third point on fault correction is, as the title of this chapter states, Fault correction, fault correction, fault correction! Make sure that you are constantly correcting your individual clients and groups. It should be considered, said in a way that is not inflammatory or confronting, and consistent. It may take some time for a client or group to get the message, but you have to continue to convey this message in such a way that they eventually understand what you are talking about.

Think about this. How often have you heard someone tell you something over and over, or you have read the same message, and it has still not really sunk in? Then, one day you will hear the same message but it may be in a slightly different way, or using different phrases and words, and all of a sudden you get it, and it is a revelation to you. Often, the phrase may be the same day in, day out and you become immune to it, and it is only when it is conveyed in a slightly different way that you all of a sudden become aware of the intention. This has happened to me many times in my life, and when you eventually get the picture, you say to yourself, "Wow! Now I get it!"

You need to practice fault correction. This is how I have done it over the years. Firstly, take a simple exercise like a "push-up". Some common faults of a simple push-up can be back not straight, head pointing down, not going all the way to the ground, and feet not placed correctly. When I write my lesson plans, I have a column for common faults, and this is where I write the faults and the phrases I use to correct them. You can do the same. The benefit of this is that during the class, when my mind is going at a million miles an hour, thinking of what the time is and what we are doing next, and assessing the physical exertion of all attending, the fault correction terminology comes straight out as I intended, and I do not have to struggle for sentences to correct errors in form. This looks natural and instinctive, but you have practised these phrases. Eventually, it becomes second nature to be fluent and concise when fault correcting. These days many instructors have their lesson plans on the mobile phone, and although I am not a big fan of people using their phones to conduct their classes, the mobile phone is certainly one means that can easily replace the hard copy paper lesson plan.

This statement may surprise you. One of the things I have noticed over the years, while participating in, conducting or observing people exercise, is the fact that I cannot remember anyone being upset or taking offence at being corrected. On the contrary, it has been my experience that people generally enjoy being told how to do things correctly, provided that some of the principles we have mentioned are adhered to. In fact, you may find some of your clients asking you if they are doing it properly as they exercise. The reason for this is, I believe, that most people want to be informed so that they can exercise as accurately as possible. The risk of injury is reduced when you exercise with good form and no one wants to be injured.

Note: I try not to touch any of my clients. Of course I have done so, but generally they have requested it, or accepted that the only way to assist or adjust their position was for me to gently place my hands on them. My main reason for not touching the client is that I want them to remain as comfortable as possible, and an invasion of someone's personal space can cause anxiety. I am a person who responds well to people adjusting my position and touching me to do so, and I come from an era where it was generally acceptable to do this, but I try very hard not to do this now as client comfort and trust are important. I am not telling you not to do this; I am simply telling you why I do not. I have a couple of mates who are fitness trainers, and they are very comfortable massaging their clients after a workout. In fact, the clients like it and request it. I choose not to do this, and it is not a part of my service. I am happy to refer my clients to those who administer sports massage professionally.

You may have noticed, a few paragraphs ago, that when I mentioned using the correct language for fault correction, I gave a couple of examples. **It is also important that, when you give fault correction or adjustments to your client or clients, you first mention the fault and then the person.** It is true that some faults are general, and you may say something like, "get your backside down, it's in the air". Clients who think they have their backside in the air will adjust, so in this instance, there is no need to mention a name. However, when giving specific fault correction, it is always best to firstly mention the fault, for example, "make sure your feet are at least shoulder width apart", pause, "Jenny". Mention the fault and then the person or people. This is a simple technique, but it ensures that others, as well as Jenny, will correct the minute you mention the fault. If the reverse were the case, the minute you name the person, everyone else relaxes and fails to listen to the correction. **Mentioning the fault first often makes a group correction occur.**

The three main things that clients mention to me that they appreciate are, firstly, keeping in touch even when their absence may be extended; secondly, that I push them as far as they can go, or at least further than they themselves would push; and lastly, that they really like being corrected and doing the exercises as accurately as they can, and with good form.

People who exercise really want to do it properly. Look around and check out any number of instructors and groups operating in the gym, or outside at boot camps, and you will always see people doing the exercises incorrectly or with poor form. There are also clients who, no matter how long or how many times you tell them or attempt to do fault correction with them, will still have bad form. I continue to try and persuade them to adjust and do it correctly, but sometimes you have to admit defeat and simply admire them for coming to exercise anyway.

When first starting out in this field it can be hard to remember everything and, of course, fault correction takes a lot of practice. It takes some time for you to remember that not only do you have to fault-correct, make sure your clients are working to their capacity, keep an eye on their safety and think ahead with the next activity, you also need to keep an eye on the time, and make sure you work to your lesson plan and timings. This is not easy initially, but with plenty of practice, you will become very adept at doing it all.

Ensure you list common faults in your lesson plan. This may reinforce in your own mind, when you read your lesson plan again, the more common faults associated with a particular exercise.

My first attempts at group and personal training were pretty good, or so I thought at the time! It is only with the benefit of hindsight that I can now look back and see that I was not the best trainer around. I can also see that I was not the worst trainer around, and while I believe that I had good control and instructional skills, I missed a lot of fault correction, because it passed me by. I could see what some people were doing incorrectly, but by the time my mind decided how to address this and verbalise it, they had moved on to another exercise. **Until I became more proficient at fault correction, I used to give general fault correction instructions at times. For example, "Okay! The planks are looking good, but we need to make sure we keep our bodies straight and head in alignment with the body."** This is a general fault! You have not actually corrected anyone in particular, but you have mentioned a general fault that may be applicable to a few attendees.

Practice your fault correction, make it genuine and relevant, and be prepared to tell your clients why you are correcting them. I often tell my clients that I want them to have good form to maximise the benefits of exercise and reduce the possibility of injury. Both the client and instructor would agree that reducing injuries is a good goal.

6. Ego is a dirty word

We are all a bit egotistical in this game, let's face it, but beware of looking too good, or talking yourself up too much.

You should always remember that it is important for you not to look too good all the time. The main reason for this is that you need to ensure that the image you portray is achievable and reachable by the average client. Someone who looks too good can actually deter clients from attending rather than attracting clients. Now, where there is a general rule there is always an opposing view, and there are plenty of people who would be attracted by someone who looks and operates under the "too good to be true" premise. Let's go back to my explanation of why you have to be careful with your ego, and make sure you have plenty of room in your classes for your clients to shine. I'll give you some examples of what I have experienced over the years.

A few years ago, I took a combined business and pleasure trip to a few countries around the world with a view to observing gymnasiums, their codes of conduct, equipment, staff, rostering systems and methods of servicing their clients. On subsequent trips, I continued to visit different countries, and have always taken some time to check out the gyms. I would like to continue doing this, but in the meantime, I travelled globally for a number of years on business and pleasure trips. Apart from some differences in equipment and training, most of the gyms look exactly like ours in Australia. Some, admittedly, are much bigger than our average-sized gym. When I arrive in a country, I touch base with a gym owner or manager and make sure they are happy for me to snoop around in their facility, and if possible I also arrange to spend a few minutes talking to the owner or gym manager. Some of these gym visits have actually been prearranged.

When I was in London, I was invited to check out a gym in the Windsor area, and when I entered the gym my first impression was that I was walking into a Mr World Contest. All the men (there were no ladies present) looked like they had just arrived from Venice Beach. I felt very uncomfortable in this gym, given my much smaller frame, and to be honest, I was a little bit intimidated. Even the receptionist looked like he came directly from the World Wrestling Federation (WWF). I left immediately and never returned. I think that gym was full of bodybuilders, and this is fine, but it did not suit me and it would not suit everyone. As a fitness provider, you need to be able to relate to as many people as you can, and ego sometimes shines through. Not everyone likes egotistical fitness instructors, or intimidating gyms or workout environments. That gym and the men working out may have been fantastic, but my perception was that the gym was full of competitive, egotistical body builders and with my much smaller frame and ego, I felt intimidated.

I have seen people injure themselves due to ego. Weight lifting is a good case in point, where you have to leave your ego at home, and lift sensibly and within your physical capability. Apart from the boot camp activities we conducted in the years I managed a gym, most of the injuries came from men attempting to lift weights that were well beyond their capabilities. They wanted to show their mates their strength, but poor form, bad technique and heavy weights can cause damage and injury. One horrific injury I recall was where a regular, middle-aged attendee, who came with his son and was very strong, ripped the bicep muscle from both tendons at the shoulder, a complete rupture that was painful and obvious at the time. He required surgery to fix the problem and stayed away from the gym on doctor's orders for about six months. It was a terrible situation for him and for us as a business. Our client was off work, so his income stream may have been affected, and our income certainly was, as both he and his son stopped coming to the gym. It may be a bit harsh to blame just ego, but it certainly played a part.

I have worked for people who have big egos, and at times their personality does get in the way of good work and client relationships. Egotistical people may be considered, perhaps incorrectly at times, arrogant and condescending. Of course, the assessment is in the eye of the beholder, and at times I have also been accused of this trait, but I am conscious of the negative image an egotistical person may portray, and I work hard not to appear this way. You know the type I mean. Often their Facebook pages and Instagram are full of their own photos, and show very few of their clients. Ego is not always negative; some people I know with big egos also have big hearts and great work ethics.

We all know of the stereotypical gym fitness instructor who cannot make it back to the office because they are looking at themselves in the gym mirrors. Perhaps this is a little unkind, but this type of character still exists, though I suspect in much smaller numbers now. I have several associates who I know attend classes with a very egotistical instructor, and they are quite happy with him and his services. As one of them mentioned to me when I suggested that they may be a part of a segment of my book, he is a bit of a prima donna, but he runs a good class, and running a good class is what it is all about.

Egotistical people use "I" a lot when they are talking, and may not fit into a team environment as well as those who are more team oriented. Selfish and self-oriented are not great qualities to have if you wish to be a good personal trainer or group trainer. You will gain more respect by being good at what you do. Present a good role model image, and let what you do, rather than what you say, be the judge of how you are as an instructor. **A boss of mine told me a long time ago that self-praise is no recommendation. I believe this now, although at the time, as a brash young apprentice, I suspect he told me this for good reason!** I have heard instructors, young and old, male and female, promoting themselves as being very good at their job. Some of them proved to be so, and credit to them, but others did not live up to their self-promotion.

As a gym manager in an average-sized gym with a great family and community focus, I always went out of my way to help the schools and learning institutions in our local area by providing positions for work experience. School children would be taking subjects including sport and recreation, and often schools offered a Certificate II or III to senior students. This is a terrific way for young adults to learn by experience if the health and wellness industry suits them.

We could only work with the school children during school hours, and because of their age, the work experience for them was often just following a staff member around and sometimes helping with equipment set-up and so on. It was important to limit contact time with clients, due to their age and their lack of experience and qualifications. Although these students were not exposed to the nitty-gritty of the industry, they often gathered enough information to decide whether to enter the industry or not.

Full-time students, on the other hand, were older, and came out of the Technical and Further Education (TAFE) system or higher learning institutions with qualifications that were immediately usable. Sometimes they were mature age students who had experienced a lot more of life and were following their dream. Some of these students had finely tuned egos. They were different from the school-based students; these TAFE trainees were almost ready to be released to the public, and we found that what we expected from them, and what they thought we would expect from them, were two different things.

Let me explain. We commenced work or had the gym operating in the morning by 5am, so when I asked students to come in at this time and observe our opening procedures, we were sometimes met with surprised looks. Some would comply, others simply would not turn up. A few would return to their teaching institution and say that the work, or the time we expected them to arrive, was unreasonable.

Now, just in case there is any doubt about this, let me tell you that whether you work for yourself or someone else, or contract out work, there will be many times that you have to get up early to fulfil your obligation to your organisation or client. Early starts and sometimes late finishes are a fact of life in our field of work. Not being able to accept this in the learning phase of your career is not a good indicator of success in the field of health and fitness.

Just a word of warning here. Most people exercise early in the morning, or later in the day or evening, because many people have to work for a living. If you are not keen to get up early in the morning, then it is a fair bet that you are going to miss out on a reasonable slice of the potential client base.

On more than one occasion, I was told by trainees that their job was to coach clients, not clean gym equipment or vacuum floors. Anyone who operates a business will tell you of the benefits of learning the job from the ground up. There will be times in a gym when the clientele is sparse and the gym may even be empty. The boss or gym owner will expect you to be able to do minor maintenance on the gym equipment, clean, vacuum and maintain the gym. As the manager of a gymnasium, I still did all those things. I believe that gym maintenance and cleaning of equipment is now covered by the teaching institutions. Essentially, this is to make sure that students are aware of the dangers of poor mainten-ance and the Occupational Health and Safety standards, as much as anything else. Although some trainees' re-luctance to carry out this work may have been a case of ego getting in the way, it would be better to accept the challenge as learning the trade and all aspects of it, and get on with it. Be like a sponge and take it all in; undoubtedly, it will stand you in good stead.

To be fair, not every student exhibited this lack of under-standing. I must admit to having some very dedicated and professional trainees at our gym. Recently, as a sole operator, I have had quite a few trainees doing work ex-perience. In my mind, they will have no problems at all becoming very good instructors and teachers. Attitude plays a big part in our success!

Another example where ego became a concern for me was with one of my staff who ran a good class but was often accused of running the session for their own benefit, and not for the attendees. On a run, she (my in-structor), would often take off and come in first without any consideration for those behind her. In other words, her competitive nature took over, and she wanted the clients to see how fit she was. **Our gym's ideal model, and one that we insisted on for our staff, was that they needed to be able to run with those who**

needed encouragement, and not take off and use the session as a personal workout. Occasionally, there may be situations where it is acceptable to be competitive, but you want your staff to be able to relate to those who need help and encouragement. Structured, organised exercise sessions are for your clients, not you. There is a fine line between demonstrations, explanations and the instructor showing off. Participating in the class is showing great leadership; you need to find the correct balance!

Lastly, a number of years ago one of my exercise sessions involved groups working as a team. We arranged the teams, before the program commenced, into five or six physically equal, capable teams who would work together. Once every week we would set a team challenge. The main emphasis of this was for team members to work together. One very fit athlete, who was actually a triathlete, found it very difficult to relate to the team, and would often go off on his own. He had to be reminded, several times, that this session was a team event. Ego got in his way, as this client found it very hard to work at anything other than top pace. Consequently, his team suffered when teamwork was required to complete tasks. Participation in individual sports breeds a type of confidence and aura that may be mistaken for ego or arrogance. Sometimes this is the case, but it could also be the focus and dedication required for such sports.

Ego is important, but it is equally important to be humble and to ensure you compliment your attendees be they in a group or individual session. It is also very important that you only give praise when it is warranted. False praise just for the sake of it is seen by most as not being genuine, and your credibility as a trainer may be affected.

Be confident, it is a must in the health and wellness game. Clients love a confident, direct, no-nonsense approach to exercise and the way it is handled. Be careful of appearing to be egotistical or arrogant as it may not be a quality that your clients and potential clients want to observe or hear.

7. Okay! Let's talk about money

In any field, if you pursue excellence, you will always have work and be sought after. Pursue excellence, not money. Rewards, including financial gain, come to those who are good at their trade.

I have a good mate who runs a very successful business. It is not in the health and wellness industry, but it doesn't matter for the sake of this chapter. He is driven and works long hours and makes a lot of money. He is seen as successful, and why not – he works very hard and reaps the rewards. I know of some other people who are not very successful. They also work hard but don't seem to be able to make much money at what they do. My successful mate not only works hard but is business savvy. He knows how to work hard and in what areas he needs to concentrate his efforts. The other people mentioned do not. Sometimes it is as simple as that. I do believe however that business skills can be taught, although some people are born as salespeople and running a successful business comes second nature to them.

Running a business is not for everyone, and you may be completely happy to work for someone else or in a gym; it is up to you. Money, regardless of how you earn it, is important.

Regardless of your knowledge, your technical ability and your experience in the field of health and wellness, or physical fitness, you will not last long in the trade unless you have a business plan and a degree of business knowledge. You do not have to be an economics master, but you do need to have some idea of how much the business costs, and how much you need to earn to support your business and produce a profit, wage or both for you and your employees.

Let me tell you about my experience of running a business. I have had several businesses since I left the Army. One was a company in conjunction with two other partners, and two were sole operator businesses. Our partnership lasted for only a year or so because we did not make enough money to cover our expenses. The initial cost of setting up your own business is quite expensive, and it may take some time to recoup this. The chance of you making a profit in the first year is slim, in fact, the number of small businesses that fold in the first three years is disturbing, but you do not have to be one of these statistics. To give you a personal insight into my first business, at times I paid my contractors or workers but had no money for myself or my family. This fact is not new to anyone who has run a small business.

Hand in hand with the payment of your staff first, is the fact that you may not always receive payments in a timely manner from your clients. You still have bills to pay in the meantime, and on more than one occasion I have had to dip into my family savings to pay staff and associated costs. This is commonly called slow cash flow.

If you have not studied how to run a business, then I suggest you undertake some research into courses that can help you understand staff wages, superannuation, workers' compensation and your insurance risk, including liability and public indemnity. It may sound simple, and in most instances, people accept that it is, but some struggle with the concept – **you must make more money than you spend, and working on how to achieve this balance can be very challenging.**

Business is pretty simple, really, or perhaps I should say the concept is simple. Particularly, when you are starting out, you have to spend a lot of money, knowing full well that it will be some time before you actually make a decent living because of any incurred debt. I always suggest that, before committing to your business, you get some advice, do some research, and work out the best way for you to make money while achieving your goals of working in the health and wellness industry.

There are people who can help you, from bank loan officers to life and business coaches, but you have to work out what the best options are for you.

If you work only part-time in this industry, and many do, then the time and effort expended in the industry is commensurate with your income. If you are planning to work full-time in the industry, then I would suggest you do all your research while working part-time, so that you are well and truly informed of all facets of the fitness industry and how these will apply to you.

I did this with my first business. I was working full-time and making a good living, but I wanted to move into another business and work for myself, so I did it gradually. The plan was to continue with my full-time employment and work part-time in the new business. I did this for a year and during this time ascertained that I could make a full-time living with my weekend or part-time work. I resigned my full-time job and started my own business. It has not always been easy, but I made a wage immediately and have continued to do so ever since, although at times it was a very meagre wage.

Full-timers can work in a variety of areas in the fitness industry, and you may even work purely on contract. An example of this may be where you contract your services to a supplier or gym and you work part- or full-time for them. You may work for several employers in a similar way and bring in a reasonable income and never see the need to work for yourself.

Just some thoughts on overheads. Building rent, gym fees, park permits, transport costs, equipment costs and replacement, maintenance, insurances, professional association fees, first aid qualifications and any other specialist requirements and licenses you need, have to be taken into consideration when you compile your fee list. All these costs should be taken into consideration when you compose your business plan before commencing business.

Once again I can give you a simple example where I conducted aerobic boxing in a very good venue that had enough capacity for up to 14 people and my rent for the building for one hour was $25. We often filled the hall, and from a simple income of $140 my rent was only $25. A neat $115 profit, you might think, but if this was the only session I conducted, I would have to take out a portion for all the above-mentioned licenses and professional requirements. Fortunately, I had more sessions and overall I made a modest living. Incidentally, I moved after one year from this council building because our classes were growing. I found a church hall in the same suburb, but the rent was $80 each night. To make the same money as I was making in the council hall, I would have to have regular attendances of 18 people. I had very good attendances at this venue, and at one stage ran a charity aerobic boxing session for over 100 attendees. So, the more expensive venue suited me and was cost-effective. **However, I had to make sure that attendances not only covered my rent but made a profit.**

At the time of writing this, I no longer have any major rental issues, as I conduct outside classes, but I do have an arrangement with a venue provider for classes in extreme weather. In effect, I have significantly reduced my rental overheads. **At the end of the day, you need to work on a model that suits you and your business.** Let me give you an insight into how I conduct my cash flow part of the business. I consider myself fairly generous, and generally believe that most people are fairly honest. I have encountered only one or two, in all my time in this business, who want to get something for nothing, and can be a bit cheeky and not pay, or not pay the full amount. I talk to them privately, and unfortunately, sometimes it can become unpleasant, but you must tell them.

My clients pay me in a number of ways. Some pay for the year upfront at the beginning of the year. Some pay me for six months, others monthly. A percentage of my clients pay by direct debit into my bank account, and this is normally done on a weekly basis, the remainder pay me cash each time they attend my sessions. I have a few who, because of their business operations or home finances, pay me when they can. I have no problems with any of these arrangements and keep track of all of them.

At all my sessions, I have a cash tin where those that pay on a casual basis put the money. Alongside the tin is a ruled-up book where they enter their name and method of payment, and 99.9% of the time this works well. Those that pay on deals enter the amount and add a note in the remarks column. This seems to work well, and although I only have a small percentage who now pay cash, it works well for those who choose this method.

Many trainers carry portable electronic payment machines, and perhaps it is because I am a little bit old-fashioned that I don't do this. I try, as much as possible, to keep my associated costs down, so no additional bank fees apply. Although I do try to embrace the electronic age and love some of the latest products and time-saving devices, I have seen many situations where faulty equipment can be a distraction, and can crash. Cash, on the other hand, is ever present, not subject to electronic signals, and convenient. More and more of my clients prefer to pay prior, with electronic transfer of funds, or even period payments for a month, three, six or even 12 months.

Whatever methods of payments for your services you choose, make sure you publicise them well,

and ensure that those who attend your sessions respect that you are running a business. Fortunately for me, I have very few issues in this regard, but keep in mind there are people who are happy to take advantage of you. These days, you can also buy computer programs that are quite economical, that will arrange your payments and keep your books in order.

Earlier, I said that it is hard work to earn a lot of money in our industry. I hope you understand that I am not trying to deter you from being in the industry, but rather to encourage you to work hard and imaginatively in running your own business. As a sole operator I have my limitations, but I do contract out some work during the year, depending on the seasonal load. I know of several local and many more non-local operators who run very successful exercise chains.

Money, and the discussions revolving around money with regard to clients, can be an uncomfortable topic, but one that you simply have to address. You will find some people forget to pay, forget to set up a regular payment system from their bank to yours, or will tell you that they forgot the cash to pay on the day. Even one or two of my small group of cash payers will turn up at class and tell me they only have a $100 note. Some will not pay as they did not get time to go to the bank, or it is off-pay week, and the list goes on. You need to develop a method to address some of these issues.

I have no doubt that there will only be a very, very small percentage of people who will deliberately rip you off. I really believe this, but sometimes you will come up against someone who tests your patience and will make you confront them about payment. Diplomacy is the best policy, and you need to talk to them. Remember, it may simply be an error on their part, and having a discussion with them fixes this immediately.

Most trainers, gyms and health clubs offer a free session or sessions, or a week's free trial. This is a great way for people to come and try your classes without committing sums of money or signing contracts.

Money is the reason you are in the business. You would do well to study methods of compiling a fee system, collecting and monitoring your income, while keeping abreast of the latest methods of doing so.

8. The awkward, unhappy or annoying client

> Your most unhappy customers are your greatest source of learning.
> —Bill Gates

If you stay long enough in the industry, there is no doubt you will have unhappy, awkward and annoying clients or customers. In any customer service business, you will find customers or clients who are hard to handle, awkward and annoying. There will be some who simply do not like you or the way you conduct your classes, and they will leave. Here are a few of my tips in dealing with some of these clients.

The unhappy client – The client may simply be unhappy because what you are providing is not what they expected. There may be outside influences, such as your client being moody, having had a bad day at work or confronting a personal issue. Also, and I hope not for your sake, it may just be their personality. Regardless of why they are unhappy, you can only do so much to

97

make them happier. It is important not to make them feel worse than they are. Ultimately, the really unhappy person will leave, and you may never find out why they left.

My best method in dealing with an unhappy client is to let it go. I do not even mention that I have noticed they are a bit grumpy, and I try to change the mood by being bubbly and energetic and providing good energy and a positive workplace for them to work out . Sometimes your client will unload their concerns on you, and you need to be careful that your exercise session does not deteriorate into a counselling session. I must admit that, particularly at PT sessions, some clients like to keep you informed of their personal situation and although I do not ignore this and keep an interest, I am very careful about providing advice and engaging in deep conversations with the client about their private life. Once again, it is nice to be interested in their well-being, but you need to keep the relationship professional, and apart from some small talk, avoid becoming a constant sounding board and provider of advice. Your job, don't forget, is to help your client be a healthier, faster, stronger and fitter person. Don't lose sight of that.

Interestingly, many years ago a member of our gym came in for a workout and stopped to speak to me about a particular current domestic polit-

ical issue. An hour later he left the gym and had not had a workout. When I apologised for holding him up, he told me, "forget the workout; I feel a lot better having had this discussion". People come to you for a number of reasons. Exercise may be just one of them.

If your client is not happy with the way you provide your services, then it would be considerate of them to talk to you about their needs and how you are not fulfilling them. However, it has been my experience that people do not like awkward situations or conflict, and many would rather just not return. Some clients will talk to you about this, and it is so much easier for you to then address the issue and come to a mutual resolution. In most instances, it may just be a matter of adjusting the exercise routine. As a personal trainer, you are in charge of the session, but often clients want a program that suits them, and you need to be aware of this and adjust accordingly.

An example may be that someone leaves because you prescribe too much cardio, and at their initial interview, it was mentioned that they did not want to do too much cardio, so rather than reminding you, they leave. Most people do not want to upset anyone, and sometimes the parting of ways may be done gradually, with the client cancelling the occasional session, and eventually just not turning up.

You will get many excuses, and sometimes they are legitimate, but the trend is to just trail off with the personal training sessions. I have heard of some clients debating with the personal trainer, and leaving in frustration simply because there is a communication breakdown. Confrontations like this are not good for you, your client or the business. You should do everything possible to prevent this occurring. Hopefully, such instances are very rare, and I have not come across this in my experience, but I know people who have.

However, having said this, I do not believe anyone should leave your services without some sort of explanation, and while most people get attached to their personal trainer and are very loyal, there may be many legitimate reasons why people leave. According to our exit surveys at the gym I managed, moving to another location was the main reason for people leaving the gym.

If you have a relationship with your client that involves regular feedback and conversations about their program and progress, most issues between both parties will be resolved.

The annoying client – This could be a client or clients who want to tell you at every session what they are going to do, rather than what you had planned. Perhaps they refuse to do the exercises you stipulate, instead selecting their own because what you have asked is too hard or uncomfortable. Next, there are the clients I call questioners. Everything you do or demonstrate is followed up by a series of questions. There is nothing wrong with questioning, but sometimes, if they had listened to your explanations or watched your demonstrations they would not have to ask as many questions. At times, this is not only annoying but distracting, particularly in a group exercise setting. Equally annoying are the clients who tell you how to do your job, and how you are not doing it correctly. Once again, these clients are few and far between, but they exist. Be respectful but firm with these people.

Those who don't listen or are talking while you are briefing the group can also become a bit annoying, especially when they ask you to explain again what you have just mentioned because they were distracted at the time of your brief. All the above can annoy not only you but also other clients in a group session. Here are some tips on how to deal with the annoying client.

Tip 1 – Be as understanding as possible. Very few people set out to distract, upset or annoy you or anyone else. In a situation where you are working with a group and being pestered with questions, to the extent where you or the group is distracted by the questioner, it may be worthwhile to say to the client or clients who are asking all the questions, "If you have a few minutes, stay back after the session and I will answer all your questions." Often this will appease the questioner, and you can get back to working your group. In a personal training setting, it is easier to manage, but the same reply also works here. I punish attendees in my boot camp classes if I think they are deliberately trying to stall or are going too slow. Most times I will prescribe a round of push-ups and this tends to fix any minor issues of speed or concentration levels. Once again, you will know your clients and who is genuine and who is not, so it becomes a judgement thing. **Sometimes, you have to be politely honest and say, "We need to move on, so I will have to get back to you on those questions."**

Tip 2 – If you have a client that likes to run the show and do their own exercises, or who changes your program to suit themselves, here are some suggestions. Provided it is not dangerous and they are getting a workout, let them go! If you are getting paid and they are happy doing their workout under your supervision so be it. I used to get all wound up about this type of client, but now I am happy for them to be like this, provided we are working towards achieving their goals and both parties are happy. Be careful to make sure you still correct posture and advice on form, repetitions and exertion levels. If on the other hand this is not safe, and the client insists on working in a way that is dangerous, you need to intervene, be firm and tell them that they need to work with you and on your program for them. Do not let clients perform exercises incorrectly or dangerously. Unfortunately, you may need to make a business decision with regard to clients who insist on doing their own exercises incorrectly and dangerously. It is not worth your professional reputation to continue. Fortunately, the instances of you becoming associated with such a client will be very rare. There are some clients who have been prescribed particular exercises or stretches to do before exercise, so it may not be a case of ignoring you, it may simply be them looking after their own bodies.

The awkward client – someone with a disability, bad postural attitude or severe physical restrictions can be a challenge to make a program for, but it is far from impossible. It is important to remember that more time may need to be allocated to this client, and that certain exercises and stretching poses may not be suitable.

Take some time to do your research and develop ways in which exercise is not only possible for the awkward client but beneficial. Fortunately, I have had the opportunity to work with people with an intellectual disability for a number of years and I have learned that more patience, and more time to explain, demonstrate and perform the exercises is required. People with learning difficulties may lack concentration and coordination skills, so one method of working with them that I have found beneficial is breaking the session up into smaller sections and having more rest times than you would normally program.

Walking is a good start, and a progressive gradual increase in distance covered may work for them. Resistance training, if possible, should be included as a way to maintain or increase muscle mass. Strong bone density is important for the prevention of falls with these clients, particularly as they age. Importantly, exercise needs to incorporate fun, as this is a great incentive for people to not only come back to exercise, but for them to look forward to exercise. Tai Chi, Yoga and Pilates are great, particularly with helping the body to maintain balance. This is crucial as we age. One study conducted by a British Authority, concluded that injuries associated with falling, for those 65 years of age or older, are usually serious and in some cases fatal.

You will be presented with awkward, annoying or unhappy clients and you will learn from them. It may be patience, or an understanding that they too want to be happy, fit or healthy. Of course, you may learn that your manner of presentation, personal appearance, personality or method of instruction is not suited to these clients. If you get feedback in this area, then you need to address this, but if it is isolated and rare, then make sure you take it on board but don't get too uptight about it. Although people leaving can be hurtful, and at times it does affect you, remember that in most instances people only leave because of personal circumstances such as a new job, changing location or moving to a more suitable time session.

The nomadic client – you will find there are people who seem to collect group and personal trainers like stamp collectors collect stamps. I am not sure of their reasons for doing this, but can only assume they feel they have outgrown their operator, or are not happy and move on to what they think will be a better fit for them. Fortunately, as with most of the awkward or challenging clients, you do not get many of these clients, but I have certainly had a few over the years. It is hard to live up to their expectations, and for no apparent reason they will move on. Sometimes they will tell the new provider that you had deficiencies in some areas. Simply do your best and don't be too discouraged if they only stay a little while and move on. I have had a few people come to me and tell me that they were unhappy with their provider. I always ask them if they passed on that information or just simply left. Remember, if you make the client feel comfortable enough to give you feedback, both positive and negative, any necessary adjustments can then be made.

Lastly, if there is anyone who is disruptive, continues to distract clients, is generally a nuisance and is intent on causing friction in your group, then you need to make a decision. I have manoeuvred these clients away from my group, and will continue to do so. This is a last resort, and you should investigate every possible way of remedying the situation before suggesting that a client leaves, as it is obviously not good for business. However, keeping uncontrollable clients is also very bad for business. I certainly have moved people on, suggesting to them that my group is not the most suitable for them. Once again, this is very rare, as in most instances clients may not only be drawn naturally to your group, but some will also naturally fall away. This old saying is very pertinent: **"You can't please all of the people all of the time." A friend of mine, who is also a regular at personal training, told me of an old Jewish saying," For every pot there is a lid"; people need to find the correct lid!**

A whole chapter on this subject may be considered a bit extreme, and while I stress that the people discussed in this section of the book are a minority, they can cause you some concern. To reiterate, Bill Gates is reported to have said, **"Your most unhappy customers are your greatest source of learning."** I agree with Mr Gates, and being forewarned is forearmed.

9. Some tips for those doing personal training

Personal training is great, but the following will help you with some of the situations that may arise. As Lord Baden Powell said when he was forming the scouting association, "Be Prepared!"

For a number of years, I did not have the inclination to conduct personal training. I have found, at times, it lacks energy, and I struggle with the thought of someone paying a lot of money for what is a "low energy" workout. I say "low energy" because, by comparison to our group sessions, personal training is lower key. I have changed my mind because there are people who only want to work one on one. It may be for any number of reasons, but they actually want to do personal training. I still try to guide them to our group sessions, but not always successfully. The reason I try to shift them to group training will be mentioned later.

Personal training is just that, personal. You make a connection with the client and work with them to help them achieve their goal. It is a collaborative effort. You devote some of your time to help and assist them and they do the same. Ideally, this is how it should work. Personal training can be quite lucrative, and one of the best means of income for anyone in our industry.

Personal training can also be extremely satisfying for you and the client, as you take their physical journey as far as you can, working towards the goal you both have set. The satisfying thing about our industry is that we often get immediate feedback, positive and negative. My experience is that personal training is only short term. Apart from a couple of my clients, most clients who I have worked with at PT have been short term, goal oriented clients. This suits the fact that most will move on once they have achieved their goal. Personal training is more expensive for the client than group training or gym membership, so this cost is a factor that restricts personal training to a more select group of people. Obviously, not everyone can afford PT. The following point is a little negative but true, and it must be mentioned. You have to be prepared for the PT client who cancels at very late notice or who doesn't cancel at all and simply does not turn up. It will depend on how many PTs you take on, but it will happen to you at some stage. Now, while circumstances at times make turning up very hard, if not impossible, you need to be prepared to be understanding at these times although it can become frustrating.

Here is my checklist for how I conduct personal training:

1. Always be punctual – this is simply a standard procedure. Clients are generally "time poor".

2. Always be well groomed and smell fresh and clean.

3. Always be prepared for your session with all the equipment ready for the workout, and a lesson plan prepared. It may not always be in print, but preparation is paramount.

4. Always present a professional approach.

5. Always follow up with good information for your client.

6. Always admit that you have made a mistake if you have, and move on. No one is perfect.

7. Always be an example with your conduct, demonstrations and explanations.

8. Always listen to your client and take note of what is hurting them or is very uncomfortable for them, and make adjustments or give clients alternative exercises.

9. Always give them feedback, both positive and negative, but in a positive manner.

10. Keep them informed about their progress.

Here is my list of things that you should avoid when conducting personal training:

1. Never criticise your client, even if they are late to the session. Talk to them and sort it out.

2. Never invade their personal space. Work out quickly what is comfortable for them and adapt.

3. Never touch them without their permission, and only to adjust their position or posture.

4. Never ask the client to do something that you cannot do.

5. Never degrade another personal trainer or client to your present client. Don't listen to criticism of other trainers from your client.

6. Never disengage from your client to answer the phone – turn your phone off before the session commences.

7. Never set them unrealistic goals. Unachievable goals will demoralise your client.

8. Never compare your client unfavourably with another client.

9. Never swear at or bully your client.

10. Never stop fault-correcting and improving your client's form and posture.

Obviously, you may not be as strong, fast or flexible as some of your PT clients, but you need to be able to do the activity you ask them to do, even if just to demonstrate it.

My preference now is to restrict the number of PTs I conduct a week. I do this because it requires a lot of energy to plot and program for a client, and to help them progress to their goal.

Personal training generates a good return financially, and I have mentioned before that money is important when you run a business. You can buy a library full of books on how to conduct your business and make money; understand that this book does not tell you how to make money specifically. My view is to be as good as you can and money will flow. Do your business study and make sure you understand all aspects of the business. In writing this book, I want you to be better at your trade; then money and success may follow. I will mention this a few times in this book because I strongly believe in it.

Back to the personal training aspect of our business. Most operators will schedule a 30-minute or 60-minute session. There are exceptions, like a mountain climb or bike ride, where you take your client on longer activities, but generally 30 or 60 minutes is the rule. I always make sure that I slightly extend these times, a little bit like the business saying, "under promise and over deliver." Not everyone in business agrees with this practice, but **I do**, and particularly in our industry. So how does under promise and over deliver work? I always give my 30-minute session attendees more than 30 minutes. You may think that this will interfere with your personal training scheduling, but if you are organised, it will not. Although I may have three or even four sessions of personal training in a row, I always allow one hour for each. This gives me time to have a snack, have something to drink, and prepare equipment for the next person. When I managed a gym, we only allowed 15 minutes between personal training sessions, so the luxury of time is dependent on who you work for and where. Our break was by all accounts quite generous.

Some other reasons to extend the session slightly are that although I ask my clients to be warmed up and ready to go when I take over at the agreed time, not all of them have done so. The warm up and stretching take time, particularly if you want to get at least a good 20 minutes or so of High Intensity Training (HIT) during the session. Also, you want your client to feel that you provide good value for money, whatever you charge, so going that little bit extra, and not being a clock watcher, may stand you in good stead for continued business. There are no guarantees in life, except death and taxes, but the better relationship you have with your client, the more likely they are to stay with you and continue to pay for your expert services.

Use your group training as a safety net for any client who cannot afford personal training after a period, but who wants to continue to work at keeping fit and healthy. It makes good business sense to keep a client, regardless of what form of exercise they are doing with you. Some associates of mine have told me they do not offer group training, and prefer only to offer personal training, even at the risk of losing a client. Getting the mix right will be one of the challenges you have as a PT. Price, time and effort are all part of the mix, and you will find that you will go through several models until you find one that suits you.

However you plan your personal training schedule, I have to say that it can be some of the most personally rewarding work you do. Seeing a client gain confidence while they improve to reach their goals is really satisfying. I will go out of my way to help anyone who is dedicated and wants to work at their goals, even if I have to schedule some sessions at unusual hours of the day to help them.

I conducted a small survey of people who attend my group and personal training sessions, asking them the qualities they expected to see in a group and personal trainer. Here are their responses:

- Committed, understanding and an eye for work-load

- Passionate, realistic and practical

- Experience, leadership and punctuality

- Participate and have a sense of humour

- Approachable and listens to the client

- Energy, inclusiveness and knowledge

You can't please all of the people all of the time, as I have written before, but in the field of personal training and group training, you should never stop trying. Clients who participate in personal training with you are paying you a lot more than those who participate in group training. They provide a good percentage of your income, so they trust you to provide them with worthwhile, relevant and expert advice and training.

Just an observation. It appears that it is a modern trend for some personal trainers to write their program on the phone, and carry this while conducting the training. I believe this can be a very poor demonstration of your research and planning skills. A professional instructor would have rehearsed the program, be able to ad lib, demonstrate, explain and perform the entire session without referral to a phone, textbook or notes. The benefit of this is total attention and observation of your client and their needs. A failure to be able to do this indicates poor preparation. I am a fan of new technology, but professionalism in the industry should be enhanced by the introduction of technology, not downgraded. A good PT knows instinctively when 30 seconds or 60 seconds is up, and it should not be necessary to carry a phone to tell them this at **every session**.

I have grown to love and enjoy personal training now, as much as group training. I have met some fantastic people who are determined and focused on being healthier and fitter. **Personal training can be a very important, financially rewarding and personally satisfying part of your business.**

10. Some tips for those doing group training

Over the years I have had some fantastic times and built great memories of my group training sessions. Recently I wrote the following on a Facebook page with a nice group photo. "I get asked a bit what I am most proud of in regard to my PT and group training business, and one of the things that I point out is the fact that a lot of good friends met at our sessions. We have people who cycle together, go on cruises together, some even lived together. Couples from our group have married, kids I took for recreation programs when they were little have come back to join us as adults, and we have helped many achieve their physical capabilities to join the defence and protective forces. We have started many careers off in this industry and I am glad we could help. Most of the people I mentioned above would tell you that while exercise is not always fun and games, it is important to have fun as part of exercise. Have more fun."

The three things that I concentrate on when conducting group training are:

1. Planning

2. Preparation

3. Practice (Rehearsal)

Now there are of course many other things such as equipment, serviceability of the equipment, do you have enough equipment, weather conditions, the time of day you conduct this class and so on, but these are things that you will come to automatically consider with experience. It is true that planning, preparation and practice will all improve as you gain more experience, but the basis of all good lessons is the way in which you approach the three Ps. You may have heard or read of the seven Ps: "Prior Planning and Preparation Prevents Piss Poor Performances." This is an old saying, and I have adapted this to the three Ps.

Planning

*The space and time you allocate to work out
exactly what you are going to do.*

1. What kind of session is this group training going to be?

2. How long will the session take – 30, 45 or 60 minutes?

3. What time do I allocate to introduction, warm-ups, explanations and cool-downs?

4. How will I collect the money?

5. How will I record the attendances?

6. Have I got all the necessary licenses, insurances and council approvals?

7. How many people do I want in the class?

8. Am I taking all groups, or just ladies, just men, is it a mixed class?

9. What age group am I looking at?

10. What kind of venue am I going to use?

Of course, the list can go on and on, and it is true that some items may overlap into the preparation phase, but generally I have covered most things you need to be aware of. After a few years' experience, the thought process is almost automatic, and the list may actually be in your head. When starting out, however, it's always best to set out your plan on paper or computer – whatever suits you.

Preparation

Where you detail how the lesson will go from introduction, to body, to conclusion.

1. Draft a lesson plan, make it as detailed as possible (you can keep these for future reference).

2. Check the plan and rewrite or amend where necessary.

3. Do a quick run through in your head, and make sure you have covered everything.

4. Check that you have the necessary equipment for the class.

I still have a folder with lesson plans, handwritten and typed, from many years ago. While some of these may be dated, I refer to them and still use them occasionally. As you become more experienced, you can and will have a lesson plan in your pocket for quick referral. Most experienced operators still refer to lesson plans from time to time, but more often than not they have the plan in their head. I strongly recommend that you go through the processes I have detailed here until you become so proficient that you do not require formal lesson plans to conduct sessions.

Practice

*Simply what you need to do to tie
everything together.*

Some of the things that you might find when you practice are:

1. Your written timings do not work, and you go under or over time.

2. Your explanations are confusing or too long.

3. The area is not suitable for what you wanted to do.

If possible, get a couple of friends to participate as classmates, and seek their feedback. Often the best-written plans do not translate into practice so you may need to readjust your program. I always attempt to do a reconnaissance of the area to be used. If you can be there at the planned time for your lesson, you can judge if the sun is a problem for you or your students, class or clients, or perhaps the noise at that time of day is not ideal. Obviously, if you have an area allocated in the gym, you need to work out the layout of the class, and how you intend setting out the equipment and clients when they come in. There are many things that you will not be aware of initially that become apparent when you practice, particularly in the location that you intend using.

Group training provides a number of challenges. For example, what are you going to do if 20 people turn up and you have only planned for 15? How are you going to adjust your class? What if only one or two turn up? How would you react to this? What you do will come with experience, but the main thing is not to panic. I know a few people in the industry who cannot handle more people than they have planned for, and it fazes them and, unfortunately, their frustration is evident, as they become anxious and flustered. This is not an ideal situation for you, so you must plan for these things to occur. You must be able to adapt, and quickly.

This is what I do if I have a circuit set up for 10 people and 20 come. I still keep the circuit, but partner people up and use the circuit in conjunction with another activity, for example having 10 people on the circuit and 10 people doing burpees.

On the given signal to change, the people doing burpees go to a station on the circuit, and the circuit people go to burpees.

Now, this is a simple solution, and one that may appear to be planned, but in fact, I simply adapt when I become aware of the numbers. I have in the past completely changed the plan for the activity that we were going to do, simply because of the numbers of people who turned up. Having a backup is essential. A plan "B" allows you to be adaptable and flexible, and if you have these in place, your class will go very smoothly. You may have some initial issues, and the program may have some minor disruptions, but you keep them to a minimum.

In a gymnasium, you have an allocated space and equipment, such as a spin room for example, where you only have a limited number of bikes. It is not a big concern because regardless of numbers your program should be approximately the same.

You need to keep control. Sometimes when energetic, happy people get together in a group environment, they form alliances and friendships. This is a good thing, and may even be why they attend; it may be the only time they get together, and they want to talk a lot. This is completely natural and something that I encourage, within reason. It is acceptable at the assembly point while waiting for the instructor, or at the gym in the lounge, but when the class starts, you need to take control and make sure your group remains switched on for the duration of the class.

This is what I do. Before any class, I call the group to gather in, and I make any relevant announcements at this time. Try to do this exactly on the allocated starting time so that you not only start on time, but you give those who arrive at the last minute the opportunity to be present. When I have their attention, I mention any relevant notes and ask if anyone is injured or unable to participate in every activity, then we commence the class. I do this in a very authoritarian way so that there is no misunderstanding about what is going to happen. Any unnecessary chatter is quickly stopped, as it becomes distracting for the other attendees. This is important! Although some people may feel they have paid their money, and want to chat through most of the session, it is unfair to the majority who are being distracted by this chatter, so you need to politely tell the offenders to concentrate on the activity. An acceptable way to do this is to ask them to concentrate 100% on the activity. Generally, most will accept this and be quiet.

Occasionally, the odd person will not. The continual offender needs to be told privately, and in a manner that does not embarrass them, that their constant chatting is distracting and you are concerned that you may lose clients because of them. It is possible that in an extreme case, you offend the chatterbox and they leave your class. This is unfortunate, but the alternative may be that you lose some of your regular class members if you do not address this. It is a fact of life that sometimes one person can be so disruptive that others leave your services. You cannot allow this to happen and should address it quickly and sensitively.

It has been my experience that people enjoy group training for the following reasons:

- Great atmosphere and energy, exercising in a group
- Competition is good and you can measure your progress among the group
- Companionship
- It is inspirational
- It is an encouraging and supportive environment
- The social aspects are great fun
- Working with a group develops relationships outside the group

The above are only some of the reasons. I am sure that you could list many more. Many people enjoy being part of a team and belonging to a group. I am sure many aspects of group training address these desires.

Group training is fun, and it can generate a lot of energy and great training results, so don't be concerned about any issues that may arise. Deal with them as they occur and make the most of your group training business. Fortunately, when most of us start out in business we have slow beginnings with smaller groups, so we tend to learn as our business grows. Group training is exciting! Fantastic feedback from happy clients is just one of the benefits.

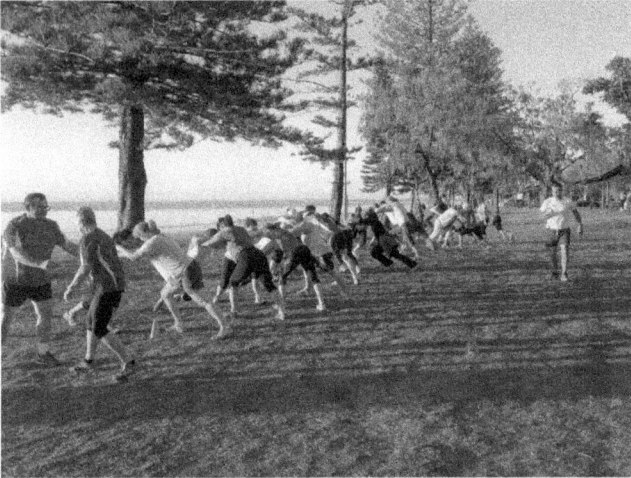

5. Group training can generate a lot of energy and great results.

11. *How I run my classes (and business, and why!)*

An insight into how I run my classes, and to some extent the general business, surrounding my work in the fitness industry.

What type of person are you? This may seem a strange question, but I believe the answer may give an insight into how you run your classes or business. A long time ago I worked in the team-building field, and a lot of that work involved outdoor pursuits. A friend reminded me one day, using rock climbing language, that people generally come in three categories: climber, base camper and puller. A climber is ambitious, always looking for new challenges and testing themselves, constantly pushing forward. The climber may upset a few more people along the way than the camper or puller. The base camper or camper is a person who is always content with their station and standing in life. They seldom push, and their ambition is limited. The camper may get on well with more people than the climber or puller. They are happy with their lot in life. The puller is trying to pull the climber down. These people tend to be a bit negative; they always see the gloomy side and may even be a bit gloomy themselves. Often, they seem to be viewed more as unhappy people, and although that may not be the case, it is a perception they project. The type of person you are will have an influence on the way you conduct your business and your approach to the business.

Some of the information I am about to relay to you is not secret, but it is unique to Tom's Law. I talk a little bit in this publication about developing your own personality and style. At Tom's Law, I have my own way of doing things, particularly with group training. My way is neither right nor wrong; it is simply my own way of doing things. I thought long and hard about mentioning these things in this book as we all like to keep a little bit of information to ourselves and while one of my chapters is called "Ego is a dirty word", most of us in the industry take pride in our work and methods. However, we remain a little protective of our own particular methods of instruction.

I currently run eight group training sessions a week, and at the time of writing this I have nine people who do personal training with me. My average attendance per group training session is 15 people. My largest group was over 100, and the smallest has been two. In addition to this, I run "one off" sessions for men, running groups and for the local council. I conduct three to four sessions a year for council, and some of these events are eight-week programs. I also host a monthly special guest breakfast with informative, interesting or famous people. The concept is to keep the breakfasts on a health and wellness theme. As you can see, I keep myself busy. I occasionally use contractors, who help me when sessions clash.

The sessions. Aerobic boxing, cross training, community program, men's only, running program and commando (boot camp), special events and activities.

Currently, I charge $10 per person for group training, $30 per half hour for personal training and $70 per hour. This information is current as at 2016. When I first started as a sole operator over six years ago, I actually charged $12 for a group session. The administrative hassle of the additional $2, plus the fact that the global economic downturn has seen the fitness industry drop prices drastically, convinced me to go to $10 a session. At present, there are gyms in my area advertising weekly fees of less than $7. A large, well-equipped gym, from a reputable chain, opened just over 1km from where I live, and charges $13 a week. Six years ago, we charged $800 a year for membership at the gym that I managed. Twenty years ago, my daughter paid $1,200 for a year's membership at a women-only gym.

The point I am making is that the Global Financial Crisis, combined with the very successful introduction of 24-hour gyms, has increased competition enormously, and subsequently membership fees have dropped, as have contracts and lengthy periods of mandatory membership.

I am aware of people who charge $5 a group training session, and a visitor from Sydney told me that they pay $17 a session for boot camp, so you can see there is great variation in fees charged.

Being confident is an excellent quality for a trainer, and this is mentioned a few times in this book. Misplaced confidence can be a drawback. I have heard several people, not all of them in our industry, tell me that they charge according to their own value and experience. That is fine, but some clients will only pay what they believe your value and experience is worth, regardless of how you see yourself. In other words, the market tends to determine pricing, not our own sometimes inflated opinion of our worth.

My rules

Everyone has rules or guidelines in regard to how they conduct their exercise programs. Here are mine:

Consequences if you turn up late. Normally, we meet at a designated spot each time and those who are late are reminded of their lateness by being given extra exercises before we start. This may be burpees or push-ups or something similar. The theory behind the additional exercise is to try to convince the attendee to turn up on time, therefore not disrupting the program. I start on time regardless of who is there, so the only thing that may really be disrupted with a late attendee is the program I have set out. The reward for being on time is no extra exercise. Now the practical side of this is that you encourage your attendees to be on time, and if not you can help them improve their overall fitness by prescribing extra repetitions.

For instance, if I have set up a circuit for 20 people and this is how many start the program, someone arriving late means that I have to adjust and rearrange the circuit. This is something we adapt to quickly, but it is inconsiderate on the part of the late client. It is true that sometimes we are made late by the circumstances of life and things that are not in our control. Regardless, I still hand out the extra work. Exercise is the winner!

The Red Shirt Brigade. You are required to wear a Tom's Law shirt or singlet to most of my sessions. This is obviously a team thing, and a marketing and advertising technique. I say most of my sessions, because there are sessions where it is not necessary. By me insisting upon this, the client is encouraged to buy our shirt or singlet. I have had clients who refused to buy a shirt or singlet, and this is fine: they simply get extra exercises to do each session. Most buy a singlet or shirt soon after joining the group to feel part of the team, and I seldom have to push this issue. Most people love being a part of an organisation or team, and looking the same is part of this process. Although it may be considered an old-fashioned technique, having your group look and dress the same has many benefits. Another often less considered reason for providing a uniform is the fact that attendees do not have to buy exercise clothes, as the choice is made for them. Without a set exercise top, some clients may not attend in appropriate clothing. Inappropriate clothing can be distracting or impractical, so providing a uniform overcomes this. Not everyone can afford the latest clothing trend, so to achieve a level playing field I insist on some uniformity among the group. This is entirely up to you, but often the team benefits are many. My group is instantly recognised wherever we train due to our distinctive uniform.

From a business point of view, it is great for marketing

and advertising. Without a doubt, it highlights our activities visually, and I am told on a regular basis by onlookers how impressed they are with a uniformly dressed, well controlled and disciplined group of exercisers.

I have to also admit that I no longer actively market T-shirts and singlets to new attendees to the same extent I did when I first started business. Generally, if the client attends more than one session, they will ask me how to buy a T-shirt or singlet. This request indicates to me their intention to stay with the group for a while, and that they also want to look like part of the group.

Don't fold your arms, rest, sit or lean. Maintain a positive posture. The principle behind this is I want to keep my clients alert and active for as long as possible during the session. All the above negative actions are indicators of resting, both mentally and physically, and I don't want this to occur. My clients know that I believe folded arms are not good for posture and resting is only to happen when I tell them. Yes, of course, we have had people faint, be sick and sit down with exhaustion, but I don't let them do this voluntarily.

Double knot your laces. Safety during training. This may seem a bit extreme, but when you think about it, you may agree with me. If you are serious about your exercise then you need to be sure that your clothing and equipment are in good order, clean, and fit you according to the type of exercise you are going to do, and that your laces are done up and double knotted. This will ensure that halfway through the marathon or circuit you are doing, you will not be distracted by having to tie up your laces. Do it right the first time. Many of us, including myself, have appreciated the fact that we can get a rest if we are working hard physically by stopping for a breather and doing up our laces. Don't allow that to happen. Double knot.

* * *

As far as I am aware, the above methods are unique to military style training and boot camps, even though some trainers certainly use incentives. My overriding reason for doing this is to keep the individual and group alert and to quickly gain control and the attention of the group when needed. There is nothing like a physical task being given to get a group to focus quickly. Sometimes, in the early morning, we can all be a bit sluggish. Additional exercises for offenders of the above, can be a great incentive to wake up quickly. Being focused mentally and physically is important, and any help I can give to an individual or group to achieve this also helps with the smoother running of the session. Sometimes, the group is awarded extra exercises for slow reactions or incorrect transition to a new exercise stand. Once again, I find the extra work quickly focuses one's mind on the job at hand.

Keep focused during training. I would love to meet the person who invented the concept of selling water to people. Brilliant! I personally have only bought water in a situation where tap water is not available. We have quite a few people who not only bring water to our sessions, but keep a hold of the water bottle during the entire program, or at the very least, have it no further than arm's length away. All this, when we have three water fountains within 200 metres of where we exercise! Fresh, clean water is available at no cost. Remove the sarcasm, and the point is that we do not break for water or to rest, and the reason for this is as follows. When we have a class that lasts for 60 minutes (at this stage, I do not conduct 45-minute sessions, and I envisage no change to this in the future), and you take at least 20 minutes from this for warm-ups and cool-downs, it only leaves 40 minutes to exercise. I want to use as much of that 40 minutes as I can to make sure everyone gets a good workout.

As an instructor, you need to provide the necessary energy to get your group motivated and moving. Once you have that energy and vibe going, the last thing you want to do is stop it working. Look at any exercise program where the instructor gives the class a break, and observe how long it takes to get the group back working to the same capacity. On a few rare occasions, I have seen people not return after a rest break, using this opportunity as an excuse to stop.

Now, don't be confused. I let people break individually, if they need to drink, go to the toilet or take a breather, but I do not break the class up for refreshments, or to have a breather. For instance, you will have, in your group class, people of varying fitness levels, and if you took a break because Mary Lou was puffing a bit, you may upset Billy Bob who is just getting his second wind. So I let everyone judge their own level of fatigue and break as they want, rather than upset the entire group. I also judge the physical exertion of each participant, and may advise an individual to break or to rest for a set. This is a very important ability that you must exercise constantly by observing the exertion levels of your clients.

At times, I call the group together to explain an exercise or activity, but I simply do not take any breaks for attendees to catch their breath or refresh.

Keep warm before you commence activity. At the beginning of the class we take off our overgarments, and put them on again at the completion of exercise. The reasons for this include having something warm to put on as soon as exercise is completed, having a corporate look with our branded T-shirts and singlets being visible and, lastly, being cooler encourages the attendee to want to get warmer faster and therefore encourages movement. There is some scientific evidence that being colder and shivering helps to burn more calories, although I suspect not enough to make a big difference.

Incidentally, a word on 45-minute sessions. I suspect that these will become more and more popular, simply because the instructor wants to reduce contact time, and most of us are time poor, so it may be that the client only wants 45 minutes. To be perfectly honest, in an ideal situation, a 45-minute session would work well, provided you did not have to do a warm-up and cool-down. If you look at even a five-minute warm up and five-minute stretch or cool-down, you are reduced to a 35-minute session, which would be fine, but in reality, this seldom happens. People arriving late can change the dynamics of your class. Time spent in explaining exercises, time between the changes of exercises, rest periods during circuits and so forth all reduce your time for exercising.

One reason why 45-minute sessions do not suit my group is because of the demographic. While we have some young people in our various exercise groups, the majority are baby boomers. Because of this, I like to take a full 10 minutes and even 15 minutes warming up and stretching. I think it is important to do this, based on their age and ailments and the fact that some people simply require a longer warm up. There is no doubt that by doing this I reduce the chances of an injury occurring during the session. Some of our programs commence at 5am, and when most people arrive for exercise, they have only been out of bed long enough to just be awake, so a slower warm up and stretch is common sense in these instances.

In a world where everything is getting smaller and more expensive, it is good customer service to provide a 60-minute session, particularly if other providers near you are moving to a shorter group session time. The choice is yours.

I try to justify every action I take with common sense, science or good management. It doesn't always work out this way, but I set out with good intentions to do this. I find that clients are always willing to accept your ideas and concepts if you have a logical reason for doing so.

I had one lady who reacted strongly to being given push-ups. Her reaction was so drastic that it is the only one I can remember, in all the years of handing out extra incentives such as push-ups and burpees. When I told her to do push-ups, because her small group that was working within our larger circuit type session was very slow, she objected violently. In front of all assembled, she told me it was unfair that she be punished for someone else's error. We discussed it for a minute or two, and she refused to do it, muttering something like she would not come back, as she left the group and the session. She did come back, and became a regular member of our daily sessions for some time after. Subsequently, she did push-ups if and when required, without question.

I have never given a punishment that I could not do myself. Interestingly enough, my exercise groups get enjoyment out of catching me out if they can, and when they do, they hand out the punishment to me. It is a bit of fun, but also highlights the fact that if you are going to enforce strict standards, you need to be able to adhere to them yourself.

Develop your own style based on your personality and character. If you do not like handing out punishments then don't do it. Work on your own uniqueness as a trainer. I have copied methods from some other instructors at times, but only those methods that I think are logical, understandable and applicable, and have something to contribute to my program and clients.

Variety. I love mixing up the exercises and sessions we do. It is not very often that we actually do the same activity, and I believe that variety is very important. I get many comments and feedback about the variety of exercises and sessions we conduct. Variety is great for the adaptation processes of the body, and helps to prevent boredom among your clients.

Some of the local trainers and their attendees see the way we run our programs as perhaps a bit strange, maybe old-fashioned and certainly unique. I don't mind that at all, because that is what sets us all apart. Work on your own uniqueness and don't ever be influenced in a negative way by other operators. Your success should be gauged on your programs and the effectiveness of the programs and the prosperity of your business.

12. Duty of Care, Obligation of Care, first aid and rehabilitation

Okay! So you can instruct. You know your stuff, are well thought of and run great sessions. **How do you react when a person in your group or personal training gets injured?** You must not only keep yourself fully qualified in the appropriate first aid requirements; you must also exhibit a confidence when dealing with injuries and illnesses when they occur, and they will occur.

A dry subject, but one that needs to be fully understood, and one that can catch you out if you are not prepared. I was told when I first started out in business, "It is much easier to keep customers than it is to recruit them". There are a number of variations of this saying, but generally, we all understand its message. Based on my experience, this saying is very true. Look at the big gyms and the way many operate. They spend a lot of time and effort recruiting members because they lose a lot of members. You often hear gym members saying that they were looked after really well before joining, but once they joined they felt they were just another number. Be aware of this, and do not ignore your clients once you have them as regulars.

A good way to hold clients is to be proficient at everything that you do. Imagine being the best personal and group trainer around, but you panic when one of your clients gets injured, and you do not know how to deal with this emergency. It will happen! Perhaps not a broken leg (it may happen, of course, and you need to be prepared), but you will be confronted with many emergency situations if you stay in this industry long enough. Learning how to handle these situations will make you a much better and more highly respected operator.

What does duty of care really mean? In its simplest form, it means that if someone is in your care then you have a duty to look after them and be professional in the way you perform your duties, and to take all necessary precautions possible, to ensure their safety and well-being. This may seem to be a tough task, but if you follow a few common-sense guidelines, it's not so daunting. In some areas, it is now called obligation of care. Semantics really – the meaning remains the same.

Firstly, let's look at the risks associated with conducting group or personal training. As a student, you were taught how to assess situations and conduct site surveys and even how to draft a risk assessment document. You need to have a risk assessment for each and every site, and at the very least you need to do a physical reconnaissance of new areas before conducting your class there. However, there may be rare times when you need to use someone else's assessment for a "one off" program, where a prior visit is impossible.

It is not possible to eliminate risk, but it is possible for you to reduce the chances of injury by careful consideration of the risks and dangers associated with the lesson you will be conducting. The area or gym space you are using may have potential dangers, and you need to consider these in your lesson plans. Regardless of your meticulous planning, sometimes accidents happen. In the following paragraphs, I have included some realistic situations and possible solutions.

Let's use a hypothetical case. In group training, you sign up a 45-year-old lady who has not exercised for 20 years, has some mild arthritis in her knees and ankles, is obviously overweight and has high blood pressure. Let's call this lady Julie for the sake of easy reference. On the first day that Julie turns up for exercise, you run your group and Julie around a very tough circuit that would be the norm for your group, but it is far too hard for Julie. In the following days, Julie finds that she is very sore, her arthritis is giving her grief, and her knees are swollen and painful. It is likely that Julie will not return to you to continue her exercise program. It is even possible that Julie may be "put off" from exercising with anyone else again, simply because of the experience she has had with you.

This is a very simple case where you, as an instructor, had a duty of care to ensure a much less painful and careful introduction to exercise for Julie. Fortunately, there was no real physical damage to Julie, but had there been, the situation may have been a bit more difficult, because you neglected to perform your job and take into consideration Julie's age and physical condition. Your attention to your duty of care responsibilities was lacking.

The above scenario is a realistic one, and similar circumstances have occurred, with me, in a group setting. You cannot always cater for one person at the expense of the group, and it is not fair on you or your group to reduce the intensity or adjust the class for one person, but there is a solution that is easy and will suit all who attend your classes. Remember that your group classes are all made up of individuals who work at different intensities, and have different ailments and pain and exercise thresholds.

The simplest way to get Julie to do all the exercises that she is able to do, and that cause her no pain, is to walk between stations. By doing this, you are making the class more accessible to Julie while ensuring that the rest of the class still gets their full workout. All attendees are doing the same circuit you set, but some, like Julie, are doing it in an adapted form. Every day I hand out instructions to our group and adapt them as appropriate. Another way of doing this is to give your instructions and then to provide an alternative with each exercise so that people have a choice. This is basic, but it is often overlooked.

At all of my classes, I ask if anyone is injured, or not 100%, at the beginning of the class. I also check on those who cannot run, just in case we are running in the class or during the warm up. This question sets up my thought processes on how I am going to adjust to make sure that everyone in the class, particularly those who are not fully fit, gets a workout.

Initially, being able to adjust your class is not easy. It comes naturally to some people, but most of us have to work at it, developing systems to help make our classes work efficiently, and keeping most people happy. I say "most people" and I mention it often throughout this book. You cannot please all the people, all the time. But you should do your absolute best to try to achieve this.

Here are two more situations that have actually happened to me, and could have ended with me, or a staff member, being in a serious situation. Both cases are related to duty of care.

As I have mentioned, I used to manage a gym. On one occasion, a member came in for his normal workout, and instead of doing his normal session, he decided to vary his set program and lift heavier weights. He set himself up on the Smith Machine and without a warm up, he attempted a very, heavy shoulder press. The weight was far too much, and came down heavily on his shoulders behind his neck. The result was a severe, spine-related injury. He missed work and had some very expensive medical bills. The gym was sued, and we agreed on a payout. Why do you think the gym was sued when the member, obviously, was performing activities that were not on his program, and lifting weights he was not capable of lifting? Well, while it was acknowledged that the member was negligent in not performing his set program, the case was put that the staff member on the floor should have intervened and corrected this member so that the injury did not occur.

As the gym manager, I believe we were not responsible, and that the ruling was incorrect, however, the gym ended up paying for a member's stupidity. The moral of the story is, you must be very careful and vigilant because serious injury can occur, and it may be because of stupidity or ignorance on the member's part, but the responsibility always falls on the operator, instructor or in this case, the gym.

Later in this chapter, I will detail how you can reduce these instances, and also the chances of you being liable in cases of injury at the workplace.

The second case involves an outdoor boot camp instructor and an attendee who injured her foot. This is an actual case and one that involved me as it was my class. However, I was taking some holidays and I had engaged a stand-in facilitator to run the sessions for the week of my absence. On the morning of the incident it had been raining, and the ground and surrounding area were damp. One of the sections of the training involved the attendees running up and down a set of wooden stairs. There is nothing wrong with the activity, as the stairs are not slippery even when wet, but when one lady stepped down from the stairs onto the concrete footing at the bottom of the stairs, her foot landed on a large leaf and this slipped, sending her crashing to the ground. At the time, it was considered simply a fall, and after the initial check by the replacement PT, the lady continued with the session, albeit with a distinct hobble. On checking with her doctor after the session, it was revealed that a bone in the foot was broken. The attendee was upset for two reasons. Firstly, the PT had not taken the incident seriously, the incident was not recorded, and the person injured was not told to get it checked medically, Secondly, the PT did not check up on the injured person later that day, or in fact at any time later.

The lady who sustained the injury did not attend any more sessions with my group, or indeed any more sessions with anyone's group, for nearly four months. To say that this client was upset is an understatement, and to be honest, the treatment of her from the moment of injury left a lot to be desired. The replacement PT was just inexperienced and downplayed the situation. Following the incident, a series of errors occurred: there was no follow-up on the attendee, no incident report was drafted, and there was no contact with her by the PT at any stage.

As no incident had been recorded, I found out about this occurrence by accident, when I returned to take over the classes after my holiday. I have since remedied the situation, but the person no longer exercises with me. It could have ended far worse. I am not being overcritical of the replacement PT, as this was a situation that could have happened to anyone simply because of inexperience and not knowing how to handle the situation. But remember, without clients, regardless of the type of health and wellness training or institute you work for, you have no business. Look after your major asset!

What should you have done in these situations?

Both of the scenarios I have detailed were actual events.

The incident in the gym could happen to anyone; it was not the fault of the gym or any instructors. The finding that we should have had supervision on the floor is valid, but an unreasonable expectation in reality. In any gym setting, there will always be people who do things that are unsafe or dangerous, and sometimes these actions are not seen. The only way you can reduce the chances of this happening in a gym setting is to have good practices and procedures in place. Yes, vigilance is important, but education of the patrons about safe practices, appropriate signage located around the gym in strategic locations, and detailed explanations of the gym rules and regulations will help. In addition, a detailed run through of all the exercises and methods of execution with every customer or client, with regard to their individual program, is mandatory. Too often the PTs will skip over the program with very little demonstration, particularly if the gym member is a regular. Don't rush through demonstrations and explanations, and offer to reacquaint clients with the execution of the exercise and using good form as often as they require it.

The second scenario is one that could easily happen to anyone. The way in which I address issues such as this, if I am the instructor, is to keep the session going by asking someone in the group to take over the group while I address the situation. In most groups, there will be people you know who can control your group training for just a few minutes. In my situation, I have qualified PTs in my group, and often we have up to five PTs attend our sessions. In some instances, they will automatically take over if they see me occupied with another client. If you have no one to do this, then select a senior or regular person to just keep the momentum for a minute or two while you assess the situation with the injured person.

I always insist on doing first aid unless the client does not want it. You need to seek their permission before administering first aid, and you cannot override their refusal even if they are being unreasonable. I carry a full first aid kit in my car, as well as a defibrillator and ice packs. Yes, I did say defibrillator, and while it is not a mandatory piece of equipment for fitness providers, I feel a lot happier knowing I have it in my vehicle should it ever be needed.[2] It is important for both the client and facilitator to acknowledge what has happened, make an

---

[2] The defibrillator is not mandatory for exercise professionals at the time of writing. I hope it will become a necessary piece of equipment for those involved in the fitness industry at a later stage. My reason for having bought one was that I have a number of senior citizens who participate in some of our group training programs. As a point of interest, I have only taken it out of my vehicle once. I had a situation where I believed a client of mine was about to have a cardiac arrest. Luckily, the machine was not required, but having it close by was a great reassurance.

assessment, remedy it and continue. There have been times where I have transported the client to a hospital for medical assessment or treatment.

Even if the injury is very minor, and the client chooses to continue, you need to be happy with that decision. There have been times where I have sent a client home and advised no further activity until they have been assessed by a doctor or medical professional. In the instance of serious injury then the session should be stopped immediately until the situation is resolved.

Addressing issues such as injury in a positive and efficient manner holds you in good stead as a health and wellness professional. While a person is injured, you do not receive the monetary benefits from their attendance, but look at the alternative. If you are negligent with an injured client, it is possible that they will never return and you will lose financially, not to mention the bad publicity that may follow your poor handling of these situations. In some rare cases, they may even try to sue you for negligence.

Rehabilitation of injuries, regardless of where the injury occurred, be it with you at an exercise session, with someone else or at work, needs to be taken seriously. I have seen too many people who do not follow their rehabilitation program through to the end experience a reoccurrence of the original injury or simply delay their return to full work or exercise due to being impatient.

How you handle clients on rehabilitation is entirely up to you. I actually stop any payments that the client may be making, and suggest that they do their rehab program with me at no cost. Let me be clear, they are on a rehab program set by a doctor or physiotherapist, not me, and their range of exercise options is limited. My theory is that they are better to stay with me and do a limited exercise program as part of their rehab while keeping in contact with their exercise associates. A person in rehab who stays away from your exercise group is more likely to get used to staying away, and bringing them back to exercise can be difficult.

Do not take first aid, your Duty of Care and Rehabilitation lightly. It may be an area that is not concentrated on enough in our training, but take it from me – it is a very important part of your professional toolbox. At the end of this chapter, I have detailed a suggested first aid kit for those who work outside gyms. At the time of writing, there is no mandatory requirement to carry specific items, and common sense would dictate that a kit should be relevant to the activity being undertaken. Incidentally, as a point of interest I use more disposable ice packs than any other item in my first aid kit.

Indemnity forms. If you take clients on any activity where they pay, and the possibility of injury, minor or severe, is present, then an indemnity form is generally signed before the session commences. The form details the possible dangers and highlights the need for people to be a certain height or fitness level, or to be fully aware of what they are about to undertake and the risks associated with such an activity. We are told by legal professionals that as a stand-alone document, an indemnity form may not mean a lot in a court of law, but combined with good briefings, good practices and safe operating procedures, the indemnity form indicates your duty of care and concern for your clients. In a gym environment, we often sent clients back to their doctors to detail their exercise restrictions, to ensure that we were working in conjunction with the relevant health professionals. This enabled us to set an appropriate exercise program for the client. You need to ensure that you are aware of the client's restrictions and capabilities. I insist on a doctor's clearance for them to exercise when I deem it necessary. I always keep the letter from the doctor on file for future reference. I have refused to let some people exercise with me, or enter our gym, because of a high blood pressure reading, and referred them to a health professional for further assessment. **The client's safety and well-being is your number one consideration. I had my indemnity form checked by a legal practitioner be-**

fore commencing my practice, and I suggest you do the same. My form also mentions the fact that I may take photos for promotional purposes. Those that are not happy with that take note and advise me accordingly.

Briefing about the possible dangers, questionnaires, indemnity forms and your discussions with the client will help you determine their physical capabilities. You need to keep their health and safety in mind at all times. Your reputation as a group or personal trainer is paramount to your business, and the way in which you treat your clients is a big part of this. A client who feels you have their best interests at heart will be much more comfortable in working to their capabilities with you.

Suggested minimal requirements for an outdoor trainer's first-aid kit

Broad bandages × 3
Band-Aid or small plasters × 1 packet
Burn cream × 1
Triangular bandage × 1
Instant ice packs × 3
Eye wash × 1
Antiseptic wound swab × 10
Sports tape × 1
Gloves × 1
Scissors × 1
Disposable resuscitation mask × 1
Sterile wound dressing × 3

13. Maintenance of equipment and hygiene

When writing this, I thought that this chapter might be one that I would skip if I were reading this book, but having worked in the industry for some time, I strongly suggest you pay good attention to maintenance of your equipment and hygiene. These are two things that are often overlooked.

Whenever we had a quiet period in the gym, our staff knew it was time to clean and maintain the gym equipment, vacuum the floor and check the toilets and showers. It was the standard operating procedure. Whether you work in a gym or have your own business, you must keep your equipment clean and in good working order. It may not be possible for you to have the latest equipment, because of cost, but you must keep your equipment serviceable and clean.

One of the biggest turnoffs for a gym is when you go to use a piece of equipment only to find that it is wet with the previous user's perspiration. This is not a pleasant experience. It is true that no matter how many signs or hygiene stations you may have in your establishment, someone will always ignore them. You must be vigilant and politely insist on policing all aspects of the gym's policy including hygiene. "No towel, no training" is a sign I have seen on a gymnasium entrance, and while you do not want to be turning patrons away, you do need to look after the majority of the membership.

As an experiment, for a year we actually provided towels to all patrons of our gym. It was a fantastic service, and one that I had seen work in a gym in Europe. The obvious problem was that we had to wash, dry and return these towels. Although we had a system that worked, we did go through a very dry period in Australia a number of years ago, and the drought conditions and water restrictions imposed because of this led us to stop the towel service.

One thing that was very successful about the towel service was that we could control the fact that a towel was being used. We supplied a full-size towel. I have seen people work out in gyms with towels that appear to be only slightly larger than a face cloth.

We were fortunate to have had a full-time cleaner on staff in our gym, and although the bulk of the cleaning was done by her, we (the gym staff) certainly had our part to play in the cleanliness and maintenance of equipment. The best thing about a full-time cleaner was that most gym members saw her in operation constantly. Some gyms only employ a cleaner on a part-time basis or in the smaller gyms the cleaning is done wholly by the gym staff.

A clean gym reduces the instances of disease and illness spreading through the gym membership, as can happen in communities where confined space and common usage occurs. Keep your workplace, your gym and your business clean, and ensure that all procedures are adhered to and that all gym members use a towel.

Maintenance of equipment is something that at times may be overlooked. This should not simply be the task of the maintenance or equipment repairer. Poorly maintained equipment can be dangerous. Loose nuts and bolts, frayed cables and rusty metal are not only unsightly but can be dangerous to users.

A maintenance schedule of all equipment, whether it is in a gym or your own inventory, should be kept and unserviceable equipment fixed or retired.

The spread of disease and germs in a team environment is rapid, and a person who is unwell and working with a team can often infect the rest of the group. It is important that they are aware that, while trying to work through their health issues is a good thing, exercise may have to take a back seat until they recover.

Despite the medical and scientific advances made in recent times, we are told that the most effective means of reducing the spread of germs is by washing our hands regularly. Most gyms now have hygiene stations situated at reception and at various places around the gym. I still prefer good old-fashioned soap and water to clean my hands once I have finished my workout.

If you are at a gym that has a sauna or a pool, you and all staff must be vigilant that these facilities are kept clean. This includes the change room and shower facilities. Apart from the obvious reasons of cleanliness and appearance, illness and infections can spread in common use areas that are not regularly maintained in a diligent manner.

If you provide boxing mitts, focus pads and so on for your clients, then hygiene with these items can be an issue. Most clients wear cotton gloves to keep their hands dry when swapping from gloves to mitts. Common use of gloves and equipment is fine, and has been a regular occurrence at gymnasiums for years, but the equipment needs to be kept dry and clean.

Boxing equipment needs to be washed regularly. This can be done, in most instances, in a normal washing machine. The gloves and mitts should be aired to dry and not put in any drying machine, as often they are made of plastic and will melt or lose shape. A few days drying in the sun are usually enough, and direct sunlight is good. I also use a spray disinfectant on my gloves before use. It is hard to completely remove the smell from the gloves, as often the sweat is ingrained, but regular washing does help to fix this.

The best solution is to encourage your clients to purchase their own gloves and look after their own equipment. This works well with your regulars, but you will always have new attendees, and they don't necessarily want to buy expensive gloves until they try the session.

I remember my childhood days at the Geraldton PCYC, where the boxing section had a wall almost full of pegs where boxing gloves and training mitts were hung up after use. The next user would simply select a set, put them on and lace them up and get on with it. The hot, wet insides of the gloves are something I always remember, as well as the heavy, sweaty smell and damp atmosphere in the area. We were encouraged to wash our hands after sparring or training. Much has changed since then, and the way we now insist on everyone having their own gloves is certainly one of the better changes.

Gym mats and floor coverings need to be washed and cleaned regularly. Perspiration, water spills and general dirt and grime will mean that you will need to clean and possibly scrub, wash and dry mats. Some gym mats are completely covered in a tough, PVC type material, and they simply need to be wiped regularly with a mild detergent and allowed to dry.

The CEO of the organisation I worked for insisted that every piece of gym furniture like benches, backrests and seats, was free of cracks and splits. As the gym manager, every week I would inspect all the exercise equipment, and if there was a hole, crack or split in the upholstery, then I would immediately get our upholsterer to come in and fix it. The theory here is that once the outside covering is no longer sealed, it quickly rips and exposes the sponge inside, and apart from looking unsightly, germs will thrive.

It is easy, in a busy environment, to forget to do regular maintenance, so to ensure that it is not forgotten, a schedule needs to be drafted and implemented. The heavier maintenance days should occur on traditionally low activity times. Often, we would schedule our lengthier maintenance of equipment on Sunday mornings, because the gym attendances were very low. If we did not finish before the gym closed at 2pm on Sundays, then we would continue to work to finish the job. The regular Monday morning gym attendees then had use of all the equipment.

Keeping your work environment clean and tidy and well-maintained is another facet of this business. In my travels around the world, I must admit that a clean, well-maintained gym is an impressive sight. It is not often clients will comment on how good a gym or facility is, but the comments on poorly maintained and not particularly clean gyms are plentiful. All the information in this chapter applies to any type of health and fitness business you are contemplating.

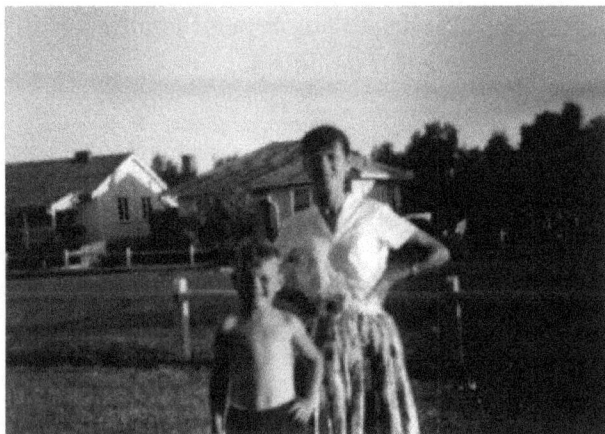

6. A family snap of Mum and me in Geraldton, Western Australia. Me in my typical dress, shorts only.

14. Interesting and important stuff

This is not the most extensive list of interesting stuff, and it is not in any specific order, but all these points are still very important.

Here is a list of interesting and important things; some may have appeared in this book and require emphasising, while others have not been mentioned at all. A book such as this has limitations, but the listed items are well worth mentioning.

The location. Where you chose to conduct your outdoor group or personal training programs is very important, and may affect the attendances you attract. It is true that a good instructor will attract a crowd regardless of location, but it can make it so much easier for you as a trainer if your area is ideal for the programs you set. Tom's Law works at a beach location called Suttons Beach at Redcliffe in Queensland, Australia, and we have the benefit of plenty of sand, good clean sea water, stairways, grass, bike and pedestrian pathways and a variety of play equipment for children and adults. All of this near our allocated permitted area. I selected the site based on all of these things, and the big bonus for me was not just the location but also the fact that we lived very nearby.

Energy. I often wonder about radio announcers or DJs and how they keep their energy levels up during an entire radio program. It is (unless a talkback show) a one-way conversation, and I suppose that is why the on-air time is only two, three or four hours. Personal and group trainers need to be similarly energetic. Let's take for example an early morning session. The instructor is generally out of bed earlier than his clients to set up, check out the site and do some rehearsals. Sometimes, depending on how far the clients have come, they are not that long out of their beds and still not fully functioning. It is the job of the instructor to quickly motivate them into the correct frame of mind and energise the group. The way in which you do this is up to you, but enthusiasm, cheerfulness and plenty of energy on your part helps you get your group motivated.

Clients, friends and customers. These are the life-blood of your business. We have discussed some types of people in chapter 8, but I didn't mention, in any depth, the great customers, clients and friends who not only like and thrive by attending your classes but also, in many instances, are your best form of advertising.

These people are some of your greatest assets, so you need to look after them. You must ensure that you keep doing the things that you have been doing that impressed them initially. You have heard the expression "If it isn't broken, don't fix it". Once you develop a good system that appears to be working, popular and effective, don't vary the formula too much. Of course, variety and change are the spice of life, and you need to look at this. Generally speaking, your regular clients will come to you because they like you, they like what you do, and it makes them fitter, happier or both.

Variety. My experience tells me, that doing the same thing all the time becomes boring and mind numbing. There are people who thrive on repetition, but most people I have encountered love variety. From a purely physical point of view, variety keeps the body guessing and the adaptation process in the body in operation. Variety also means that we are trying new things and the body is being challenged physically and mentally. Make sure you incorporate variety into your programs. I find that providing a greater variety of exercises and challenges also gives some people in our group the opportunity to shine where they may not normally. A good example is that, from my classes, I run an annual skipping challenge and competition. For the last few years, we have had people in their 60s winning sections of the competition. In fact, the skipping challenge tends to favour the slightly older clients in my groups, and I can only deduce from this that skipping played a bigger part in their childhood. It is fair to say that I have had a number of clients come to me from other providers, with the common complaint that they did the same thing all the time. Keep this in mind and introduce variety into your training.

Your fitness. You may be surprised and thinking, why does he mention the fitness of the instructor? Well, be surprised, but I have observed fitness instructors who not only did not look like fitness instructors, they were not particularly fit. Not every instructor is the fittest, strongest or fastest person in their group. I have quite a few people who attend my sessions who can outrun, outlift and outlast me, but I am fit enough to be able to do everything I ask of my clients. The quickest way to disappoint your clients is for you to ask them to do what you cannot. Yes, we all know the typical, middle-aged coach with a slight paunch who stands in the middle of the field with a whistle strung around his neck, barking out orders. Our industry is different. Coaches are there to pass on their experience, and to make sure their athletes work to schedule. They have to time, correct, record and encourage their stable of athletes. Their job is not to be as fit as their athletes or to compete with them. Athletes are finely tuned, highly motivated, and have been working in their field for some time, and generally, know the exercises and stretches they should be doing.

The normal fitness client is looking for you to demonstrate, correct them, and to inspire and motivate them by example. The only way you can do this is to present a fit and healthy model who can demonstrate and perform in a way in which you want your clients to emulate. One of the fastest ways to lose respect from a client is to ask them to perform exercises and repetitions that you cannot do. Once again, I see this from time to time in the industry, and while there will be times when you are incapacitated or injured, and a simple explanation is all you can manage, this should be the exception, not the norm. A degree of common sense is required in how you read this. I have people in our group who can do the splits. I cannot, so obviously, I would not expect my entire group to be able to do the splits.

Your appearance. Although we have mentioned your appearance in another chapter, it is important to highlight this again, in more depth. When I first started out in the industry, we were told to make sure that we were clean shaven and well groomed. We have moved on now, and although clean shaven is not a requirement and stubble is very popular, you must be well presented, neat and clean. The required clothing is simple but needs to be clean, and it is preferable to look clean and fresh at the start of your session. Although your clients will seldom comment on how you are dressed or presented if you follow these guidelines, they will certainly mention your appearance if you are unkempt. **Never**, never turn up to conduct a group training or personal training session if you are under the influence of, or smelling of, alcohol. Smelling clean is simply a reference to body odour, which affects all of us, and is just another facet of personal hygiene.

Your example. It is easier to say than do. You need to concentrate on being the best example you can possibly be. Some common complaints that I have heard from clients over the years include the instructor being biased towards certain attendees. It is hard not to be impressed with those in your class who work hard and achieve certain goals. Be just as observant and vigilant towards those in your class who struggle to achieve a chin-up or even those who have difficulty in stretching during the warm up. Remember, you would not have a job without those who are new to exercise, so make sure you are fair and completely unbiased in the way you interact with your clients. I would like a dollar for every time I have heard a disgruntled client say "they seemed to concentrate on their favourites", "we were ignored", or words to that effect. It is a fine balancing act to make sure you give the right amount of encouragement and compliments. Make sure you do not exclude any client, and work out a way to get to every client for corrections and encouragement at least once during a group training session.

Your demonstrations. Although mentioned before, in another chapter, I cannot emphasise enough how important it is that you demonstrate the exercises in the best way you can and with the best form. You will find that your demonstrations will be closely observed and copied. Make them as best as you can, and get plenty of practice by yourself, or even with others observing and fault-correcting to help fine tune your demonstrations. Never give your clients an exercise to perform that you cannot do. The main reasons for this are because you cannot demonstrate it properly, and secondly, unless it is a specific exercise for an elite athlete, you should not be giving stretches and exercises to your clients if they are too difficult **for you** to show them exactly what you want them to perform.

Humour. The use of humour can lighten the load of every person in your group or personal training session. Humour should be natural, not forced or nasty in nature for obvious reasons. A good joke or a quip that breaks the tension, can often help the situation and make the session just that little bit more achievable. In chapter 9, humour was mentioned as a quality that was desirable, for a group or personal trainer, by some who participated in my survey. Use your natural character to develop your own style and approach. If you are naturally funny and can inject some humour from time to time into your sessions, then this will only add to your reputation as a well-rounded health professional. Don't force humour; it seldom works and can be very awkward.

Punctuality. It is worth mentioning again that you provide a great example as an instructor. Clients will leave if they have to wait past the published time for a session to start, and naturally enough, the same will apply if you go over time with your sessions. Punctuality is expected, so you should start your sessions on time. People are generally time poor. They have allocated a set time to exercise and cannot, and will not, tolerate tardiness with instructors who do not start and finish on time. I believe it is important to start your session at the correct time, and this is paramount. It is less important to finish on time, but you need to tell your clients when the time is up. A good example of this is where you are doing a specific challenge at your session, and some people are still working on finishing the challenge at the set finishing time of your activity. Tell them the time is up, and give them the opportunity to leave or finish the challenge. Most people have been late for one reason or another, and this is generally well accepted, but a continual offender will feel the consequences.

I know some clients who have left a PT because they were tardy starting on time. There is no excuse for being late. Your gear and equipment needs to be set up and ready to go by the designated starting time. Late attenders need to be aware that you will not wait for them. In fact, in my group sessions, late attenders are punished with push-ups or burpees, as discussed in chapter 11.

Today I was speaking to a potential client who told me of her personal trainer who was constantly late to their sessions, and the most disappointing thing, from this client's point of view, was that the personal trainer was asking top dollar for his services.

15. *Working with children*

Working with children in Australia is generally accepted as unique, and specific modules and courses exist to educate instructors in this field.

Children are a joy to work with in most instances. I have had experience with those just starting school, to young men and women about to be launched into the workforce, children from affluent parents, to those who are not as fortunate and even those who have become (according to the various agencies) disenfranchised. I have had extensive experience with children with learning difficulties, and those who have come from the wrong side of the tracks. Children are often the most challenging group of people to work with, and I think this is because children will give you immediate and honest feedback. Children, in many cases, have not developed a great sense of diplomacy, and quite often are blunt in their feedback.

You cannot fool children for long, and any attempt to present boring, tiring and repetitive ex-

ercises will be met with a general lack of enthusiasm on their part. Keep them interested with dynamic challenges, and you will have a much better chance of keeping them participating.

Up to eight years of age. I have had the privilege of working with many schools, assisting in the facilitation of exercise and activity programs for their students. My opening statement about children being a joy to work with is extremely accurate with this age group of children. They are obedient, willing to please, and generally well regimented in the ways and procedures of the school. These children present some challenges but, overall, they are willing to listen, and they are always excited.

Assistance is normally required from the school or institution depending on the size of the group, but I remember fondly the great times I have had working with children in this age range. The most memorable thing about this age group is their enthusiasm and willingness to please. I can still see now the smiling faces filled with excitement and anticipation.

I have been caught out with at least one program I wrote and conducted for a school with pre-school children. I overestimated the degree of control over their bodies that children of this age have, and some of the exercises were too advanced. Although this is specifically about children, the lesson I learned here applies to every group regardless of age. Be careful about the challenges you set, and keep in mind the capability of the individuals and groups, their ages and stages of development.

I find this group a lot of fun. For a number of years, I ran a children's program we called KIDZONE and KID-STUFF for children 4 to 12 years of age. Initially, we called this an activity program, simply because "exercise" is not always particularly attractive to children or their parents. I created fun activities that involved exercise, from mini obstacle courses to bike rides and bike challenges, cubby house building, swimming activities, billycart races and so on.

Working with children in Australia now requires the provider to have some additional checks. A police and security check is now a mandatory requirement; this is commonly called a Blue Card. You apply through the Federal Government to obtain a Working with Children Permit (Blue Card). You will also need, as with any exercise practice, insurance, professional qualifications and in some instances, depending on your operation, a suitable and approved venue.

My involvement now with children's programs is mainly through the local government programs as a contractor. However, I still need to maintain all the appropriate paperwork, often more than is required

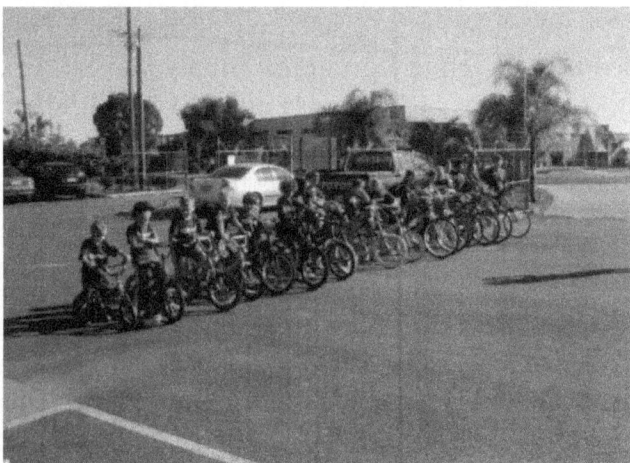

7. The KIDSTUFF team lines up with their bikes ready to head off on another activity.

for training adults. The main reason I only work with children seasonally and through council programs is because it became difficult, on a weekly basis, to compete with organisations such as Little Athletics, AFL's Auskick, Life Saving Nippers, a variety of martial arts programs and the many sports competitions being held around Australia every weekend. The programs I have mentioned are extremely well organised and geared to large numbers of children, and it is hard to compete and be financially viable. Fortunately, my programs with children were cost neutral. I did not make any money on these programs, as I was offering all children the activities, including those from a lower socio-economic background. The program worked as a promotional vehicle for me because it was part of my involvement in the local community.

In my estimation, weekend programs for children are very competitive, but not impossible. I believe there is an opening and a larger market for after school care exercise and activity programs. There are at least two of these programs operating in our local area, and they are very well attended.

Some parents like to be involved with their children's activities, and others will seem a lot less interested. There are parents who cannot attend due to work or other commitments. You will find that if you engage the parents, then they will help you with control and assist you in most areas of your activity. Occasionally, you will encounter parents who, regardless of how much effort you put in and the activities you devise, will not be entirely happy. My suggestion to you is to keep these parents informed on what you are doing, how you are doing it and the benefits of the activity. In my experience, the awkward parent is rare, but you do need to be aware of their presence and devise a way to accommodate them. After all, we are working with their children.

Don't attempt a children's program unless you are happy to work very hard. I have found that devising, planning and implementing children's programs to be difficult at times. You have to consider the child, the age group and what activities are suitable for a particular age, as well as making the activities engaging. This is not always easy, and as I have already mentioned, it can be more difficult than conducting programs for adults. **If you like working with children, and have no issues with hard work, then it is extremely rewarding. Kids provide an energy and rawness that is refreshing, educational and surprising.**

16. Communication skills, marketing and advertising

To some, communication, marketing and advertising of your business will be the most important aspect after your skills and qualifications. How many events have you missed because you simply didn't know they were on?

One of the best communicators I have ever met is Gerrard Gosens. Gerrard is a blind athlete, motivational speaker, businessman and great friend of mine and my family and an amazing man. Gerrard and I met many years ago when we were both involved in other organisations. He was with Guide Dogs Queensland and I was in the Australian Army, and together with a large support and running crew, we ran from Cairns to Brisbane collecting money along the way for Guide Dogs Queensland. Gerrard had, and still has, a very high public profile, and he is the best person I have ever seen at exploiting his profile to the maximum. Well-educated, a fluent and influential speaker and a great athlete, Gerrard has no difficulties even today at getting great publicity for his events and exploits. But then if you have flown a plane, run marathon distances, competed in triathlons and attempted to conquer Mt Everest, and you are totally blind, you may find yourself being a highly sought after speaker. Gerrard also appeared on our small screens nationally a few years ago when he was selected to compete in the Australian version of "Dancing with the Stars". Not one to let the grass grow under his feet, I am proud to call Gerrard, Heather and their family friends of ours.

Being able to communicate effectively will help you to run an efficient business. It will allow you to be a better employee and help you to understand your clients. The best operator in our field cannot reach their potential unless they have mastered the various, and ever changing, methods of communicating their assets and skills to their clientele. This includes client progress and feedback. I have never had any client give me negative feedback when I have contacted them to ask, from their point of view, how the classes were going.

It was not that long ago that my daughter suggested to me that I needed to start a page on Facebook to help promote my business. As someone who has not grown up in the technological age, Facebook, emails, and the host of other electronic vehicles including the mobile phone were not things that I completely understood or was familiar with. I have seen the mobile phone in its various forms develop over the years, and I can use a computer, but compared with the children and youth of today I am a novice. Even my very young grandchildren can show me a thing or two about computers and tablets, but I am not completely useless.

I now have a Facebook page and a web page, and I am on Instagram. I can use a mobile phone effectively, but I am far from an expert, though I can get by. For those things that I do not understand, I engage my daughter Robyn, who is very tech savvy, or I pay for expert advice. More about this form of communication for marketing later in this chapter. I am more adept at using some of the not so modern means of communication – not that I consider myself brilliant at it, but I continue to work to be a better communicator at work and home.

Verbal Communication. This is something we use every day, and although we seldom think about the way we communicate verbally, from a business point of view it is very important, particularly how you communicate verbally with your clients. Communication skills – Speed and rhythm is very important, as it is for a race caller or sports commentator. The way these people speak and communicate is highly descriptive, and can build expectation and excitement. Using your voice in a very effective way as a trainer is a great asset. If you are not good at this, then develop it. Practice the use of words, phrases and the tone and RSVP of your voice. An acronym that I have used and I find particularly useful, in regard to voice training, is RSVP.

R Rhythm. The rhythm of your voice and the way you use this can be beneficial in our trade. You can set the cadence (pace or timing) to make sure that everyone is working at the rate you intended. Take step-ups for example. You may want a speed of 24 steps to the minute, so you can set that pace with your voice and the rhythm you use, "up up, down down, up up, down down".

S Speed. The speed at which you speak or give instructions can be a distraction. If you speak too fast, some things you say may be missed. If you speak too slowly, people become impatient. Choose a speed that is easily understood. You can also use speed to increase energy levels, and if you decrease your speed you can slow down an activity. Learn to harness all the variances of speed in your voice.

V Volume. If you speak too softly, then people cannot hear you. If you speak too loudly, it may become annoying, not only to the group but to other people not in your exercise group who may be nearby.

P Pitch. This is also called the tone of your voice. Have you ever heard an annoying voice to the extent that it really distracts you? I recently was watching some cartoons with my grandchildren, and one of the characters had a voice that was very gravelly and deep. The voice was so distinctive that it annoyed me to the extent that I could not watch the cartoon. The voice literally hurt my ears. In our industry, we have some instructors who scream. This is not desirable, and adjustments should be made to ensure that the pitch used is acceptable to the majority of the participants.

RSVP. Easy to remember.

What is your message? I have covered how to impart your message; now we need to ensure that it is easily understood. Sometimes what we think is clear and concise may not always come across to our clients that way. I have no doubt that despite my best attempts to convey a clear and concise message with good demonstrations, there will always be a percentage of people who do not understand the message the way that I intended. This is a fact of life, and you can only do your best. Try to keep the explanations short and accurate and remember the old saying, "a picture tells a thousand words". Use demonstrations wherever you can.

Don't overexplain. I get told, from time to time, that I give too many instructions. Work at being short and direct with your verbal communications skills; sometimes less is more.

Non-verbal skills. We are told all the time that our non-verbal communication makes up a good percentage of our communication skills. This is one of the reasons that many businesses like to have videoconferencing. Instant non-verbal feedback is important, and our manner, facial expressions or arm and body movements tell more about how we are feeling than just verbal communication does.

For example:

- A speaker is giving their address and you agree with the statements they are making, so you nod your head in agreement.

- You show your happiness when you see something pleasant on the TV and you smile, or you grimace when something nasty comes on.

- Your facial expressions often give immediate feedback before you can follow it up with your concerns or comments.

- When presented with disturbing news we often shake our head in disgust with an action similar to nodding "no".

In our field, you can see the feedback almost straight away when you are briefing a group of people. It is great information, and you need to be aware of the feedback and how it may affect you and your session. It is equally important that you can respond quickly to the feedback you get.

A person suffering may need to rest longer than the rest of the group. A general response of boredom from your group is an indicator to change the activity or to inject some fun or variety.

It makes sense that you need to be adept at understanding these signs and learn how to get feedback from your clients in different situations. During the class, you will be constantly checking for injuries and exercises that are proving difficult. You will be looking at the perceived rate of exertion, seeing the enthusiasm and excitement in the faces of those enjoying their exercise, and seeing the pain or lack of enthusiasm etched in the faces of others.

Keeping in touch with your clients. I have mentioned this several times in the book, but it is worth going into more depth about how important it is.

As I have stated, **the best operator in our field cannot reach their potential unless they have mastered the various, and ever changing, methods of communicating their assets and skills to their clientele. This includes client progress and feedback.** This statement is one that everyone should take note of. Failure to communicate well will adversely affect your business.

Report back to clients. "I hope you have pulled up well after your initial session with us on Monday, Julie. Some people have reported sore abdominals after this session, and it is perfectly normal. Should you have any queries, please do not hesitate to call or email me. Looking forward to seeing you on Wednesday." This is one way to let your client (who has attended their very first session with you) know that you are appreciative of their attendance and that there may be delayed onset of muscle soreness.

Modern means of communication. I work with and co-operate closely with some younger personal trainers who are miles ahead of me with the modern forms of communication. They are faster, can problem-solve quickly, and understand all the various forms of electronic media. As well as being a good operator with all the skills and qualifications necessary, you will be left behind by your competitors unless you embrace and exploit the modern means of communication you have at your disposal.

I use Facebook, Instagram, emails, send out a weekly newsletter and have advertisements on local radio. I also have banners and sandwich boards set up in my location, and I have leaflets and business cards that I hand out freely and frequently. Sometimes we publish a leaflet and do a letterbox drop. I also have a regular spot on community radio.

We even advertise through our corporate look. The

group T-shirts, singlets, hoodies, caps and even the car stickers that I hand out freely, all help to advertise me and my business. You will be surprised how many people notice these things on the road, not only locally but overseas. I have someone who comes over from New Zealand from time to time, and they exercise with us. Believe it or not, someone reported back to me that when they were in New Zealand, they spotted a Tom's Law car sticker. The following is another story about car stickers by one of our highly thought of friends and an attendee at Tom's Law.

A client, Donna, was telling the story the other day about how good it is to have a Tom's Law sticker on her car. I was in another conversation but heard the chuckles, and when Donna mentioned how good the stickers were, I thought, "there is a catch here, somewhere", and there was. I went back to Donna to get the full story, and here it is. Apparently, some time this year Donna visited Sea World. Those of you who know the major theme parks in Queensland know that the car parking area is enormous. Donna has a very popular make, model and colour of car, so when Donna left the theme park in the afternoon, it took her a little while to find her car because she had forgotten where she parked it, but the Tom's Law sticker did the trick. Now, that in itself is not all that funny, but in my mind, and in the minds of the people Donna was telling, perhaps it was the image of a mature woman wandering up and down the parking area looking for her car. I don't mind admitting that I have done similar things many times. Anyway, if you tend to lose your car, just ask me for a Tom's Law sticker; it may save you some time!

Several trainers I know, who are very good at what they do, have little if any contact with their clients outside their sessions. Of course, years ago we did not have the almost immediate means of contact that we have today, but if you don't use whatever technology you have at hand, you may be left behind by those who embrace the modern forms of communication. I would be the first to admit that keeping in touch with your clients between sessions is very time-consuming. However, in an extremely competitive field like ours, you need to embrace and master every possible way to keep your clients informed. Once again, you are the master of how you run your business, so it is up to you.

Part of my opening statement on this chapter is worth stating again. **I have never had any client give me negative feedback when I have contacted them to enquire, from their point of view, how the classes were going.** Every client I have contacted with this enquiry has been appreciative of my concern and glad I contacted them. Find a way to show your clients your concern, and make sure you use all the communication skills and means you have at your disposal to keep your clients happy and well informed.

I ring, email or message my missing clients on a regular basis to ask why they have not attended our sessions. Obviously, I do this from a genuine concern point of view, as it may be that I have offended, upset or mismanaged them. Of course, I am concerned as to why they have not attended our session, and sometimes it may be because they are on holidays, are unwell, or indeed it could be any number of reasons, including dissatisfaction with the instructor or some of my attendees. I try to do this every Friday, rain, hail or shine. This doesn't mean that I have always been happy with their response as to why they have not attended, but any negative response is also good feedback. I can then address the issue or at least be aware of it. You may want to keep computer records of attendances, and I use a combination of manual sign-in and computer entry to ensure I keep up with who is attending, and who has dropped off the system.

You need to work hard at keeping up with the best methods to serve clients, the latest trends, means of communication and exercise options, and the list goes on. The beauty of our business is that you will never stop learning, and the more you learn, the better you can provide the services your clients want. We are all looking for the edge that will help to make our business as successful as possible.

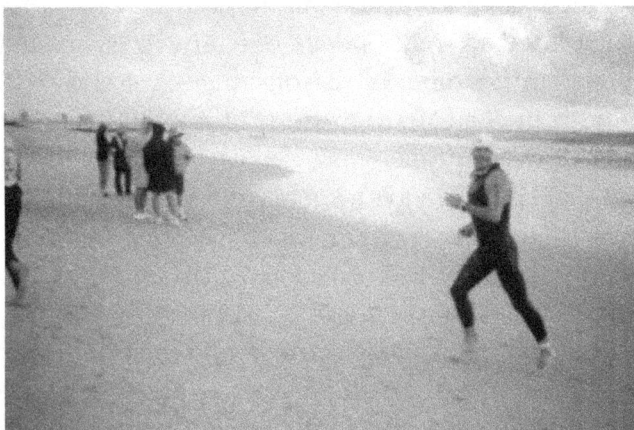

8. Coming out of the water at my first big triathlon at
Mooloolaba, Queensland, 1997.

17. The last word

During the process of writing this book I became aware of many things I have not mentioned. I am happy that in such a small book I have crammed in as much as I possibly can to hopefully inform, educate and perhaps even inspire you to be better at your chosen profession. At the very least I hope that I have convinced you that this profession is a very rewarding one, and I hope that you continue to strive for improvement. **The rewards are enormous.**

Consistency is very important. Let me give you an example of how we strive to be very consistent. Working in the outdoor industry in Queensland subjects you to all the elements. Our summers can be stormy and our winters cold. The extremes are not as drastic as in some countries, but client comfort and safety is a concern, so although we do not like to do it, we may have to cancel some sessions due to the weather. From a Tom's Law point of view, we only cancel because of health and safety. By that, I mean that bad weather is an individual perception and one person may be convinced not to attend a fitness class due to the weather where another person assesses the weather as acceptable and will attend. From my point of view, we keep consistent by only cancelling sessions in extreme weather due to health and safety.

Perhaps this is an obvious title for the last chapter in the book. I am taking this opportunity to mention some things that have not been covered so far, and also to review some of the more important things I believe will help you to become a much better personal trainer. A book with every possible pitfall and good practice for personal trainers and group trainers would be so big it would be hard to carry, but we have covered a lot of relevant information in this book.

Learn from others. Every day, when you see trainers operating, observe them and what they are doing. Sometimes, it may be obvious that you are watching, but try not to distract the instructor or class. You will learn so much from this. I have never believed any one instructor, however well-educated, practised and experienced, has a monopoly on good instruction or customer service. You will see some things that are not ideal, and it is up to you to decide if you believe that by adopting some of those practices it will improve your business. Often those who are working full-time in the industry have achieved a level of professionalism that perpetuates their business. Those with doubtful practices and operational glitches seldom stay in full-time operation for long. There are exceptions, of course. Most businesses operate the same way: sink, survive or thrive.

There is very little in our industry that is original. Most businesses in the health and fitness industry tend to follow fitness trends. Seminars, conferences and educational forums keep most of us informed, and these events provide a vital function in keeping us well-educated in the latest trends in our industry. Observing fellow operators can be just as fulfilling and educational. I have no doubt that some operators have observed my practices and implemented them into their program. In fact, as a mentor to many young operators in the industry, I know this to be a fact. Equally, I have used many ideas and sets that I have seen others in the fitness industry use, and by doing this we add another dimension to our own operations.

I have never stopped learning, and I hope I never will. If I could pick one thing that I admire about many of the youngsters who I see joining our field of employment, it would be their enthusiasm for knowledge. Those who continually seek knowledge are already a long way towards making a fine contribution to the health and fitness industry.

Keep in mind that you may encounter some very experienced people from all walks of life in your practice, including doctors, physiotherapists, chiropractors, nurses and paramedics. Surprisingly, you may also have, in your group, people who previously were qualified in the fitness area. These people have a wealth of knowledge, and you should keep this in mind. An example of where it has helped me is when I have had to deal with an injury a number of people in our group, who were training with me at the time, have been capable of and have often taken over the group while I tend to the injury or apply first aid.

Treat everyone the same. You will come unstuck if you do not treat every person the same. As has already been mentioned, a personal or group trainer must treat every client with respect and in a kind and spirited way. Of course, there will be times when you are not well thought of. You may have insisted that a client work past their comfort zone, but favouritism and preferential treatment of clients is unprofessional, and your business will suffer if you are not aware of this.

Don't be too protective of your business and try to expand your network, even among those you may see as competitors. I believe we all have our niche market and I have never experienced mass migration from one PT or group trainer to another. Yes, from time to time there will be the transient client as I have mentioned before, who will flutter from gym to gym and instructor to instructor.

Be heartened if another operator copies or uses a similar marketing strategy to you as those who copy you are paying you a big compliment. If you find instructors using your methods of instruction, games and so on then also be heartened. I have found that by embracing the local PT community in my area, we can work in co-operation on some common projects. Seldom do we promote similar events, because we have different demographics. One may concentrate on Mums and Bubs, the others may be young males, another may be a combination of both, and some are boot camps or boxing classes, so variety prevails and the clients in our area are the winners.

Engage the local community. At Tom's Law, we run some free classes. Every week I hold a free session for the community as a genuine gesture of my intention to try and help as many people as possible. I support and sponsor local community radio. Of course, the audience is limited but importantly, it is local. My group supports local fun runs, and we are well known in the area for doing so. Get involved in the community. Every year we select a local charity and run a few events to help them out. In 2016, it was the St John Ambulance of Redcliffe.

A word on nutrition. Although I can suggest a healthy eating plan and am qualified to advise on nutrition, I choose not to. The reason is simple; my knowledge is limited compared to that of a nutritionist or dietician, and I therefore prefer to refer my clients to a full-time professional in the field. It is up to you, and I do know of many PTs who not only advise but send meal plans and eating programs to clients. Nutrition is a specialised area, and I am not keen to advise my clients when people who are more highly qualified than I am are readily available. Diabetes, coeliac disease, food intolerances and allergies are much more prevalent now than in the past, and specific dietary advice should be sought.

Although many PTs align themselves with businesses that provide bulk powders and supplements, I do not sell, advise clients to use supplements or promote them. I have recommended the odd multivitamin, and zinc or fish oil tablets, but the choice remains with the client, and I do not pressure them into taking supplements as part of their exercise program. Research and a chat with their local general practitioner will generally assist clients to make the correct decision about the supplements they may or may not need.

My reluctance to sell, promote or recommend supplements is my personal choice as I do understand that there may be a time and place for supplements. My qualifications are limited when it comes to supplements and nutritional advice, so I prefer to refer my clients to more qualified experts in this field. Let me quote you the paragraph that refers to this in my nutrition workbook for the Diploma of Fitness.

> The aim of this module is to provide instructors and trainers with skills and knowledge that can be applied, to enable them to work with clients with specific nutritional needs. The module provides information on a range of metabolic conditions which require clients to modify their food intake. It should be emphasised that instructors and trainers would work in association with dieticians when providing services to these clients.

I have a local dietician/nutritionist and sports physiologist who I refer clients to and work in conjunction with.

Sometimes, you may come across a family member, good friend or even a mentor in the industry. If this is a person you trust, then you should listen to them and their advice. I have several trusted friends who give me good advice, tell me when I am going off track and boost my confidence when I need it. I will often pass ideas by them, and they have the knack of being able to tell me straight if something is not going to work. They are tactful, mature and experienced, and their advice is very valuable. These friends are businesspeople and their experience in business has helped them, and I appreciate them mentoring me.

A hope this book opens your eyes to more of the industry and gives you some assistance as you

work in this field.

I have had to learn, even in my 50s, that working on a gut feeling or impulse is not always a good way to operate. I have had my share of triumphs and successes, but a more measured way of doing business is to research thoroughly, investigate as much as you possibly can, seek the opinion of family and friends, then act. I tend to be a "it is better to beg for forgiveness than seek permission" type of person, and it has held me in good stead, but as I get older, I am certainly a bit wiser, and I have a more measured approach to life and business.

I hope you find your way in this industry, love what you do and become successful. Perhaps you are working in the industry at the moment, and want a change of direction or to start up your own business. Whatever you are doing in the health and wellness field remember this.

This is one of the most positive fields you could possibly want to work in. Helping people achieve their wellness aims, assisting them to be healthier and happier, and being part of the overall plan to reduce illness and promote healthy living is commendable.

Good Luck – Tom.

Testimonials

I had the pleasure of being introduced to Tom 13 months ago when I had my first training boot camp down at his training facility at Suttons Beach.

I had not done any training or exercise for at least 15 years and had let myself go – I had been an Australian Rules player in my younger days, so I had been exposed to high level training and fitness methods over the course of my sporting career.

Tom put me through my paces, accessed my fitness level or lack of it, and then explained in simple terms what he was going to do to assist me get back on track.

This is a key element to any good trainer – being able to access the trainee and ensure that they work to their limits during each session. Tom is one of the best at this task. His eye for his charges is something that can only be gained by experience. His Army, fitness knowledge and life experience shine through in every single training drill he conducts.

This book gives an insight into the man 'Tom Law' and the methods that have guided him throughout his life in his passion of health and well-being through fitness, and I cannot think of anyone with more experience, professionalism, understanding and resourcefulness in his chosen field. He has turned my life around. Thank you Tom.

Michael Glover, Redcliffe, Queensland

I was very fortunate to witness the work ethics and determination shown by Tom Law as a fellow employee at Pine Rivers Shire Council. Tom held a difficult position and at times a thankless one but in true Law spirit did not shirk his responsibilities.

I also have great respect for Tom by the compassion and encouragement expressed to me while recovering from Cancer in the year 2000. Tom was manager of Spectrum Gym at the time and without his input my recovery would have suffered. Thanks my friend.

I have continued my gym activities since and believe this at the age of 73 has attributed to my healthy lifestyle.

Tom's determination has helped many, many people live a better life and for this he should be commended.

Tom, thank you my friend.

Alastair McTavish, Murrumba Downs, Queensland

There are so many things I have done since training with Tom that I never thought I would. Tom changed the way I view myself, my body and my life. Tom is someone I will forever hold deep in my heart and his success is from a will to help others. He has always been community focused and worked some sessions for free. Tom is a true gentleman, a hero for our country with his honourable military service and hero to our community for all the lives he touches and paths he creates for people to follow.

Shendelle Harrison, Regional Manager – Central Qld & Whitsunday, BT Advice Dip. FS (FP)

Almost four years ago, my family and I were walking along Sutton's Beach when we noticed a guy in a bright yellow shirt conducting a children's fitness session. I was so impressed how he had the kids captivated all the while they didn't realise they were exercising, laughing and giggling. Then I came across his sign Tom's Law and took his flyer. Later that day I called Tom and booked myself and my husband in for a group fitness session. We were new to the area and thought this would be a great way to meet new people while trying to get fitter. We are large people and were a little hesitant about going along to the group but that didn't last long as we noticed what a diverse group of people were there. All levels of fitness, ages, personalities, strengths and weaknesses. Walking away from the first session I had an extra spring in my step as we felt great. Tom guided us through the session showing us how to do the exercises correctly by doing the exercises with us and not barking orders, as we had experienced with other PT.

By the second session we both knew this was the way to the next healthier phase of our lives.

In almost four years, I have never been to a session that has been the same. Tom's knowledge of fitness is amazing as I've watched and learned the most simple of things that I never thought I could or would ever undertake. I have achieved so much in a short time because of Tom's dedication to all he teaches. I believe his service and experience in the Army is what has given him the discipline and loyalty that he displays always. What I love most about Tom's Law is the fact that it's not just fitness it's all about a healthy lifestyle. Through Tom's guidance we can all live healthier and happier.

Thank you Tom for all you do, you have certainly changed my life.

Sally-Anne Stubbings